THE
TANGO
EFFECT

THE
TANGO
EFFECT

Parkinson's and the healing power of dance

KATE SWINDLEHURST

with contributions from John Connatty and
Ellie McKenny

unbound

First published in 2020

Unbound
6th Floor Mutual House, 70 Conduit Street, London W1S 2GF
www.unbound.com

Text design by PDQ Digital Media Solutions Ltd.

A CIP record for this book is available from the British Library

ISBN 978-1-78352-803-5 (hardback)
ISBN 978-1-78352-804-2 (ebook)

Printed in Great Britain by CPI Group (UK)

1 3 5 7 9 8 6 4 2

For Andy, Tom and Kathryn as promised

*With special thanks to Emily Rawlence Bilmes and Louise Ells
for their support of this book*

Those friends thou hast, and their adoption tried,
Grapple them to thy soul with hoops of steel

— Polonius, *Hamlet*, Act I, Scene iii

Contents

Introduction

The Tango Effect explores the impact of Argentine tango on my experience of Parkinson's disease. It begins with a tango lesson which became a short story* and then an article,[1] written in collaboration with Cambridge Tango dancers and teachers Ellie McKenny and John Connatty. Soon, we found even an article wasn't enough; this book is the result.

Ellie McKenny was particularly interested in investigating the creative possibilities of tango. Having trained as a clinical psychologist, she first experienced tango personally as an escape from the emphasis on judgement and analysis in her training and then in her working life. When she became a tango teacher, working with adults with learning disabilities or ill health alerted her to the way that – for the duration of the dance at least – identities linked to disability or illness, psychologist or client, teacher or pupil, could disappear.

Tango teacher John Connatty shared my journey from its outset. Keen to understand 'how it feels for you to

---

* For the short story 'Touch', see the Appendix, page 161.

overcome that bit which has gone on the blink', he was not only ready to encourage his student but committed to the process of discovery: 'Maybe your brain can develop a way around the block... Maybe the music somehow puts your brain into a less self-conscious state from where it is possible to float around the problem. We can be pioneers!'

The Tango Effect records what we discovered during our year-long investigation into the effects of my tango habit on living with Parkinson's. In many ways these effects are remarkable, although those who have some knowledge of the condition will not be surprised by links between exercise and well-being. Some readers may already be familiar with research that matches aspects of Argentine tango with strategies for improving quality of life for people with Parkinson's. Still, many I speak to are new to the idea and react with astonishment, excitement and a desire to know more, in that order. If you are one of these people, this book is for you.

If you are already a dancer, you will know that Argentine tango differs from what many regard as the 'classic' ballroom tango made famous by Hollywood. I think some of my friends imagine me high-kicking round the floor in red satin and fishnets. Occasionally I do dress up, but tango itself is something separate from glamour and might equally be danced by an old lady in a cardigan or a student in torn jeans, both with heart-stopping beauty. Others picture an intensive aerobic fitness class, zumba with heels. The tango I am engaged in is not about classes or performances and is improvised rather than choreographed. This is social tango, danced with one partner at a time, usually as part of a gathering with other dancers. It relies absolutely on communication between those involved.

To *aficionados* and onlookers alike, Argentine tango is the epitome of passion. I've attempted to convey something of the experience of that passion as well as a taste of the extraordinary complexity and fascination of the dance, its history, its music, its poetry. Inevitably, there is so much more to say. If you would like to know more, there are several excellent books on the subject, some of which are listed in the bibliography on page 177.

The word 'passion' doesn't sit easily in the same sentence as 'Parkinson's', and for those with the condition, communication itself can be difficult. You may find yourself slow to respond to others and have difficulty concentrating. Your speech may be slurred. Sometimes the voice becomes so quiet it is hard to hear. If depression is a feature of your illness, you may tend to withdraw from social interaction until you become locked in a bubble of your own making. Tango can burst the bubble: challenging the tendency to isolation in its reliance on the unspoken connection between partners, it offers a rare experience of intimacy for the Parkinson's dancer.

The profile of the disease differs from person to person, so you won't find a comprehensive explanation of each aspect in these pages. For me the first hints that something was wrong were a right arm which hung uselessly at my side while running and when my elaborate italic handwriting shrank to a cramped knot. My GP gave up the search for a tape measure and improvised with a piece of string, which he wrapped round my upper arm. Was he looking for signs of muscle atrophy? And why did he ask me to walk the length of the surgery while he watched?

There was no explanation, so I was still holding on to illusions of a trapped nerve when the neurologist offered his diagnosis. Ten years later, I ticked most boxes on a checklist of symptoms and there had been some deterioration, but it wasn't much. In this way, and in the relative mildness of many of the disease's features that I was experiencing, I was one of the lucky ones. Still, once you have Parkinson's, there is no going back. You may not get worse, at least for a while, but you will not get better.

Or so they say. Is there, in fact, such a clear division between illness and health? Despite the sense that your battle with disease begins with the diagnosis, you have, of course, been living with it for years. Once diagnosed, medication may make you feel better. If you are fortunate, it may enable you to live relatively symptom-free without side effects. And you may discover for yourself other routes to well-being: yoga to counter stiffness, perhaps; cycling as an alternative to walking; or Argentine tango. In our investigation we were keen to examine that apparently firm line between well and ill, and excited by the possibility that tango seemed able to persuade the damaged brain to work as if it were undamaged. Perhaps it could even reverse the progress of the disease?

The Tango Effect is an intensely personal account that echoes what the science is beginning to tell us about the healing power of tango. While neither self-help book, triumph-over-tragedy nor misery memoir, it tells a story that we believe demonstrates life-changing possibilities and will be of interest to medical professionals and the academic community as well as those living with Parkinson's.

It's eight years since the start of our collaboration, and our story isn't finished. There is certainly room for more research into the benefits of dance for those with Parkinson's, especially in relation to quality of life, rather than the more easily measurable gains in motor function. Meanwhile, there are new dance opportunities opening up for those with the condition locally, nationally and internationally, as well as rapid progress in medical research[2] into early diagnosis and more effective treatments, leading eventually, perhaps, towards a cure. For now, we look to our tango family for love, inspiration and support.

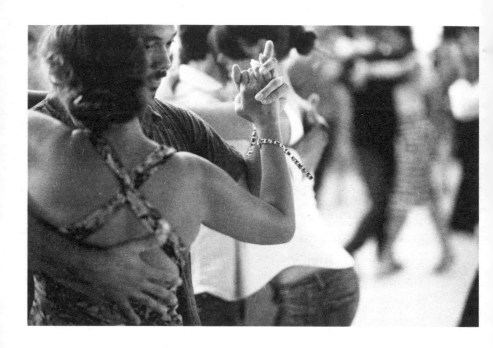

Prologue

A Thursday night: a man stands in the doorway, another in the darkness by the far wall. Tonight there are lots of students – beautiful young women who glide with such poise, and even the awkwardness of the beginner is captivating. Next to me, in the line of chairs along the edge of the floor, an older couple, here every week; dogged, unsmiling, they dance only with each other. Voices, laughter, the whirr and hiss of the fans. On every table, glasses of water; I am one of the few with a glass of wine. I sit at the back, aware of the niggling tremor in my right arm, anxious about the imminent challenge of getting smoothly to my feet. On the floor, a scattering of dancers, waiting to see what the next set will bring. Now those first notes – raw, urgent, unmistakable: the sound of Pugliese's orchestra. I also have been waiting. I know exactly who I want as a partner. He is on the other side of the room, too far for eye contact but I look directly at him anyway, tilting my head slightly. He nods. I struggle to my feet as he walks towards me and we step into the procession of circling bodies. He lifts his left arm, the hand open for my right hand. I place my other hand on his shoulder, lean into his chest, muscle against muscle, his arm on my back. We breathe. I listen for his intention. When we move, we move as one. No shaking; no halting or stumbling. There are only these: the imperatives of the music, now fast, now slowing almost to a stop, suspended; the connection, unspoken, heart to heart; and the astonishing gift of grace.

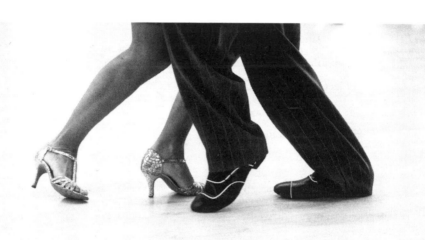

January:
New Year, New Beginnings

Date: 1 January

From: John

Subject: Improvers course

Hello tout le monde,

By now you will obviously be suffering tango withdrawal symptoms so it might be a good time to raise the following: I have been approached by several of you from the last improvers' course to run another similar one, so I am canvassing support. I currently have time on my hands so I could offer a course starting mid-Jan, probably Saturday mornings and Sunday afternoons.

Please let me know if you are interested – if I get enough positives I'll put together a schedule. Don't forget we restart at St Paul's on Tuesday 4 Jan @ 7.30pm.

Regards, and wishing you a Happy New Year!

P.S. Private lessons available.

The first lesson: a wintry morning in Cambridge, though the sun shone. One stop on the train. No one was there to meet me as we'd arranged, but I knew where to go:

around the corner, a gravel drive. I rang the bell and waited, nervous. Once inside, a woman I didn't know sat on the opposite sofa and chatted as I changed my shoes. She said I was brave, coming out for a private lesson. I blurted out the Parkinson's story. 'Oh well, you can tell John,' she said. 'He's a good listener.'

He was. Sympathetic but without fuss, he went ahead with the lesson without trying to minimise the condition in the way that others often do in their attempt, I suppose, to encourage me or cheer me up. The right arm I explained needlessly, as it alternately jerked and stiffened to its own rhythm. 'We can work round that,' he said. Already it felt as though we were a team.

Although I hadn't danced for a while, I wasn't new to tango. In a way, this had become part of the problem. Ten years earlier I had found myself in a small class of beginners in a remote town in north-east Cumbria. An odd assortment of shapes, sizes, aptitude and aspiration, we practised walking like panthers while our instructor, Francis, a self-styled Argentinian from the Scottish Borders, modelled the task. I remember feeling both absorbed and baffled. Over the coming weeks, we collected moves – *ochos* and *ganchos*, *barridas* and *boleos* – showing off our party tricks at every opportunity. The longer we danced, of course, the more we realised how little we knew. Still, for a while the novelty and excitement carried me through. I had become a dancer! I remembered the excruciating awkwardness of the occasional church disco I was allowed to attend in my teens, the determinedly solitary nature of sports I eventually came to pursue – swimming, distance running. Here was an activity that was, if not for team players, at least enjoyed in company.

For some months I even had a regular dance partner. Philip, a charming Buddhist painter, lived with his parents in Carlisle. We met at the beginners' classes and danced on Tuesday evenings in a tiny upstairs room overlooking Devonshire Street, the high ceilings, long windows and the lamplit traffic outside creating the illusion that we were tucked away in a corner of Buenos Aires. Monday nights, we practised in Philip's parents' garage, which was floored with slabs of chipboard. Frequently I stopped mid-turn, distracted by a stack of tins – peas or tuna – that his mother was hoarding against who knew what emergency.

Things change, though: for Philip, a disgruntled girlfriend and thrombosis; for me, exhaustion at work, difficulties with balance and a growing tendency to wobble on the dance floor. One morning, running on the treadmill at the gym, I noticed in the big mirror in front of me that while my left arm was behaving normally – nice and relaxed, at waist height – my right arm was just hanging there. I wasn't particularly worried, and didn't think to connect this with my increasingly spidery handwriting or to falls I'd had while running through the woods. A colleague persuaded me to visit the doctor – perhaps she recognised the signs? The GP certainly did, although neither prepared me for what I was to hear from the consultant: 'I'm ninety-nine per cent sure you have Parkinson's,' he said. 'I'll leave you on your own to think about that for a few minutes.' I remember having a little cry and then going back to work in time for the last lesson of the day, a cover lesson for an absent science teacher. I sat in the lab, itself foreign ground for an English teacher, stunned by the news and trying to make sense of this new world.

In tango, our teacher was replaced by two real Argentinians. I learned more but danced less. My confidence shrivelled. I was older, less well. Eventually I managed to secure early retirement from teaching on grounds of ill health and talked myself up sufficiently for a first visit to Argentina, organised for members of the tango class by our new teachers. Despite some wonderful moments and the support of the group I travelled with, I found the dancing more intimidating than pleasurable. I have a photograph of myself taken in Club Gricel in Buenos Aires, with Hernan my 'taxi dancer' – a paid partner for the evening – and his beautiful girlfriend (both barely out of their teens and a full foot shorter than me) smiling for the camera. I am leaning sideways wonkily, explosive with panic.

At home, nothing eased the difficulties of dancing with Parkinson's or my dwindling confidence. I knew that tango was reputed to be helpful to people with the condition, but I was often disheartened enough to consider giving up dancing entirely. If it hadn't been for my writing, I might have done just that. Incredibly, or so it seems now, I had made that first visit to Argentina in complete ignorance of the country's history, in particular the horrors of the 'Dirty War', when up to 30,000 people were kidnapped, tortured and killed by the military dictatorship. Back in the UK, I began to find out. At about the same time, now that I was no longer tied to the classroom, I was keen to write more and looked for a writing course to support me. After a term on genre-writing in Newcastle, the punishing 100-mile drive on Wednesday nights was proving too much. Instead I applied for a place on the MA in creative writing at Anglia Ruskin University in Cambridge and persuaded my brother to let me sleep on his couch for the year, hoping to rent out my Cumbrian cottage.

From Cumbria to Cambridge; from Cambridge to Buenos Aires: the extraordinary, dark chapter of Argentina in the 1970s had stayed with me and the MA provided the framework for me to grow the fragments in my mind into my first novel. The prologue – in the voice of one of the 'disappeared' – arrived almost whole. The next 80,000 words took more coaxing. But support from Arts Council England enabled me to make a second trip to Argentina, specifically for research. Once there, how could I leave Buenos Aires without at least trying to dip a toe in the tango water, even if most attempts were spent shivering on the side of the pool?

Nine months later, while back in Cumbria for the university holidays, with the first draft of the novel finished, I was invited to the Christmas milonga in Carlisle. Somewhere I still have my dance card, blank where the list of partners should be. I remember a long evening's watching. Nonetheless, by the end of the night, my friend and dancer Nancy's plan for another tango visit to Argentina's capital had grown into an expedition of twenty or more – and I was on the list.

So here I was, just outside Cambridge on a Thursday morning at the start of the new year, with everything to play for. I felt the muscles at the back of my neck and across my shoulders start to soften. My right arm settled. I remembered to breathe. Afterwards I left full of hope. More than simply encouraging, John seemed ready to take on the whole Parkinson's *thing* as a challenge. This might actually work. We agreed on an hour's lesson a week for as long as I could afford it, in the run-up to my Argentina trip at the end of March. In between, I followed the group course, John and Ellie sharing the teaching, and attended the weekly milongas, where I danced with others from the classes and with John, who made a point of dancing with every individual student. He was attentive, courteous and interested. That these qualities seemed unusual is perhaps a measure of my low opinion of myself at the time. He left me feeling both special and equal. Something in his manner invited confidences as well as confidence. When I told him one dancer had spotted my tremor and jumped to an accurate conclusion, he said, 'Does that matter?' For me this felt huge: did this mean it was OK to be who I was, how I was, rather than struggling to keep the condition hidden? Perhaps this was the beginning of learning to live with myself more comfortably, as the actor Michael J. Fox discovered after he 'came out' about his Parkinson's:

Nothing more, nothing less, just exactly who I am.[1]

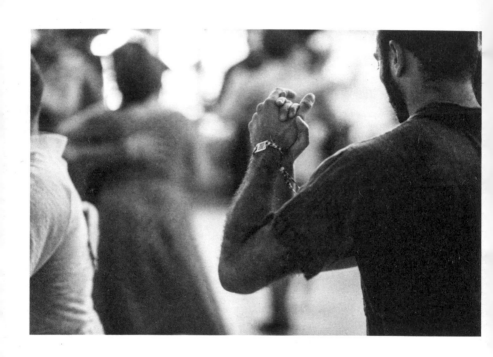

February:
Parkinson's

Ellie: I've been thinking — how about supporting Kate to write a paper about her experiences?

John (laughs): That's good — Kate wants the three of us to write a book!

In 1817, Dr James Parkinson published an essay on the 'shaking palsy', which he also called *Paralysis agitans,* describing symptoms he had observed in a handful of individuals while walking through London's streets to visit his patients. After his death, his name was given to the condition that he identified. The son of an apothecary and surgeon, he worked from his home in Shoreditch. He was a champion of the underprivileged and a medical all-rounder, as well as something of a pioneer: he was the first in English medical history to write about peritonitis, for example. I imagine him pacing the streets of the East End and wonder what first alerted him to the signs of the disorder he discovered. What would he have made of these gentrified streets today: the hipster beards, the trendy galleries, the bars and restaurants? He had an April birthday, two days before mine.

The disease that bears his name is a chronic and progressive neurological condition, sometimes misleadingly described as a movement disorder. Parkinson's involves the malfunction and death of dopamine-producing nerve cells in the area of the brain called the substantia nigra. The chemical dopamine is a neurotransmitter that sends messages to the part of the brain that controls movement and coordination. By the time the symptoms become noticeable, it is likely that there has already been an 80 per cent decrease in dopamine production. In the UK, of a population of almost 67 million, figures for 2018 estimate that 145,000 people, or one in every 460, are living with Parkinson's, with two new diagnoses every hour. By 2025, the total is likely to rise to 168,000. In the United States, the current total is around 1 million, with an estimated 10 million cases worldwide.[1] The cause is unknown, although most explanations suggest that heredity and environmental factors may contribute. There is currently no cure, despite the often-heard comment that it is 'only a matter of time'. Still, hopes for the future[2] include potential breakthroughs in earlier diagnosis by using brain scans and blood or breath tests, and reprogramming brain cells to reverse the symptoms. There are various treatment options, and newer ones involving inhalers or deep-brain ultrasound therapies are becoming more widely available. However, most current treatments don't slow, stop or reverse the progress of the disease and come with unwelcome side effects.

The symptoms of the disease are most obviously a tremor, slowness of movement (bradykinesia), rigidity and 'postural instability' – a tendency to lose one's balance and therefore be prone to falling. However, there is no normal profile and not everyone will experience all of these. The symptoms can appear in any order, although they often begin on one side of the body and slowly get worse. Most cases come to light in adults over the age of fifty (I was fifty-four) but one in twenty adults diagnosed with Parkinson's is under forty. There are several other movement-related effects; those I experience include impaired dexterity and coordination, and cramped handwriting. Increasingly I find I am prone to 'freezing', suddenly unable to step or turn, as if my feet are glued to the floor. In addition, many people with Parkinson's suffer from constipation and several studies suggest that the condition may actually originate in the gut rather than the brain. People with Parkinson's may also have problems sleeping and concentrating, and experience emotional and psychological difficulties. Fatigue and depression have been particularly challenging for me.

A growing body of evidence demonstrates the benefits of exercise for those with Parkinson's. Aside from the range of anecdotal evidence on the positive impact of exercise on mood, flexibility and so on, research has focused on its effects on the brain. Dr Kim Gerecke, now Associate Professor of Behavioral Neuroscience at Randolph-Macon College,

Virginia, has investigated ways in which exercise can protect the brain against neurodegenerative disease. Studies with mice[3] found that three months' daily exercise protected their brains against a neurotoxin that mimicked the effects of the disease. Reducing the time span or frequency of the exercise reduced the protection. A similar investigation[4] suggested that, since the neural pathways are present and undamaged (unlike in stroke victims, for example), the brain can be retrained to produce more dopamine or, where dopamine-producing cells are already lost, to manage with less or work more efficiently. It appears that exercise may bathe the damaged neurons and circuits in the brain with nutrients that make them sprout new connections and survive for longer. Studies in California[5] found that people with Parkinson's who took exercise moved more normally than those who did not. This suggests that, in certain situations, the neuroplasticity created from exercise may actually outweigh the effects of neurodegeneration. Now researchers at Newcastle University are developing movement-based computer games for systems like the Xbox, incorporating increasingly complex programs using sound and visuals to help make exercise more effective for people with Parkinson's.

From the range of exercise options, dance is becoming widely recognised as a useful therapeutic tool. The Dance Psychology Lab at the University of Hertfordshire is well established and committed to ongoing research into the physical and psychological effects of dance on people with Parkinson's, and several British and American dance companies now offer classes for this group. In Wimbledon, south London, for example, dancer and choreographer Simone Sistarelli teaches weekly 'Popping for Parkinson's' classes, while in Broomfield, Colorado, the Art as Action collective offers a 'thriving multi-faceted program' drawing on an eclectic mix of jazz, modern, contemporary, hip-hop and ballet under the 'Reconnect' banner.

Tango in particular is becoming recognised as a force for change: in a preliminary study at Washington University St Louis, on the effects of tango on 'functional mobility' in Parkinson's disease, the writers commented on 'emerging evidence' that the basal ganglia – the parts of the brain particularly affected by Parkinson's – are 'specifically involved in the control of dance movements'.[6] In a further study, researchers Madeleine Hackney and Gammon Earhart compared the effects of Argentine tango and American ballroom on a sample of fifty-eight people with mild to moderate Parkinson's. They suggested that several step patterns in tango actually mimic the rehabilitation exercises designed to target the 'freezing' problem, and may serve as external 'cues'.[7] A system of 'cueing' – replacing the missing internal cues with external stimuli – is widely used in the rehabilitation of people with Parkinson's to target gait difficulties, slowness of movement and freezing. According to the study, the degree of difficulty is crucial: tango is essentially a 'multitasking activity' that demands 'dynamic balance and involves turning, initiation of movement, and moving at a variety of speeds'.

Building on these early studies, Dr Hackney has continued to explore and promote the therapeutic potential of Argentine tango.[8] Currently Assistant Professor of Medicine, Division of General and Geriatric Medicine at Emory University School of Medicine in Atlanta, Georgia, Hackney is also a research health scientist at the Atlanta VA (Veteran Affairs) Center for Visual and Neurocognitive Rehabilitation. A former professional dancer, she has developed a form of 'adapted tango' with modifications in steps and in the embrace, which she believes is best suited to those with Parkinson's, and has trained instructors to teach classes using this model. Recently she co-authored a study which found that after twenty dance sessions, people with Parkinson's improved in gait, balance and motor control, and in muscular control and coordination.[9] She believes that tango may also help improve spatial recognition and quality of life, and is now working with MRI scanning to investigate the effects of tango on the brain, believing that the music and dance help to promote long-lasting improvements in neural connections.

The mental and physical requirements of tango are matched by the emotional demands it makes on dancers, particularly in the area of confidence. To step onto the floor into a close embrace, you have to believe in yourself, in your capability and your worth as a partner. It's a big ask for any dancer. Conditions such as Parkinson's chip away at self-esteem. There is nothing attractive about its characteristics, and it is difficult not to become preoccupied with what you can't do. Simple tasks (fastening buttons, putting on socks, getting change out of a purse) become tiresomely challenging, walking downstairs an exercise in mind over precarious matter. In tango, surrounded by other, more beautiful, more experienced, younger, able-bodied dancers, where does a dancer with Parkinson's find the courage?

During those first few months of the year, as I began to trust him, John helped me to rebuild my confidence. We quickly moved beyond steps and techniques – his belief in my ability to improve felt like a promise: this was a battle we could win. His unqualified support reminded me of psychologist Carl Rogers' belief that 'unconditional positive regard'[10] is a key factor in enabling human beings to fulfil their potential. According to Rogers, like his family's winter supply of potatoes[11] putting out shoots even in the dark basement, we are constantly striving to become what we're supposed to be. In the warmth and light of John's regard, how could I possibly not grow? And, incredibly, tango wasn't just making me feel better. The increase in my personal confidence was matched by a steady improvement in my general health. Somehow, tango was replacing my fatigue with energy, transforming rigidity to fluency, translating tremor to stillness, restoring grace.

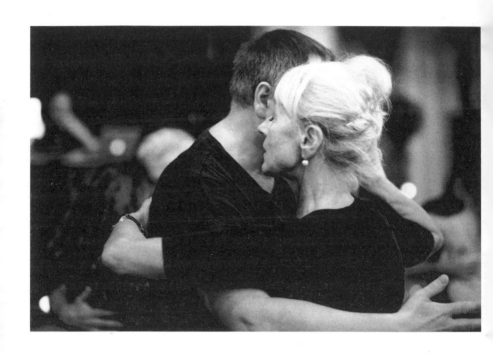

March:
Argentine Tango

For me, tango is about communication, about listening and responding to each other and to the music, and about the community context of the milonga. The better the listening and response from the pair, the better the dance, the better the connection. In my opinion, this connection works best when there is acceptance of difference combined with a readiness to suspend judgement, a commitment on both parts to fit together as one. This is when the real tango medicine kicks in: two people with limited expectations of themselves and each other agreeing to move together to the music, finding and being themselves.

— Ellie

Tango is not always seen as beneficial for health. In fact, author, teacher and tango *aficionada* Christine Denniston describes it as a 'contagion'.[1] Certainly the tango obsessive is a familiar figure to the initiated: first to arrive at every milonga and last to leave, driving miles through the night to get to and from another dance opportunity, discussing the intricacies of the dance or, for female dancers, the merits of a particular heel height with anyone who will listen. It has become – or has it always been? – a dance of extremes and contradictions: while in its early years polite society frowned on its association with the brothel, today ardent fans emphasise its almost spiritual qualities. Some regard it as the ultimate in machismo, others as a liberating experience for the woman. It has been claimed variously by the avant-garde and by traditionalists. It is notorious for the predatory figure of the older male on the lookout for a younger female partner, although I have also seen it danced beautifully by preteens and by couples in their eighties.

Part of the power of tango to captivate such a wide and committed audience stems, perhaps, from its extensive roots. Popular accounts of the origins of tango focus on the end of the nineteenth century. Single men from rural Argentina and from Europe flooded into Buenos Aires in search of work, in response to government-sponsored schemes to provide manpower for agriculture and for industries now booming following railway expansion. Alone in a strange city halfway between a glamorous European-style capital and a lawless frontier town, the men turned to each other for comfort, making their own music, dancing with each other and with any women they could find. However, their music and dance evolved against a background of earlier settlements, as the new immigrants met the strong music and dance traditions already established: Moorish and Arabic influences from the

Spanish communities, such as flamenco; the Afro-Cuban habanera; and the music and dance of the central and west African slave heritage, particularly from the Congo. In fact, this may be the derivation of the name 'tango', which in Congolese means a dance or a 'place for dancing', although some still favour the Latin (via Portuguese) verb *tango*, from *tangere* (touch). As in Montevideo, in neighbouring Uruguay, European migrants added Italian opera, the waltz and the polka to the musical mix.

Grainy photographs from the early 1900s show men in work clothes and big hats looking into the camera as they sit outside a building, or dancing in couples in the street. My favourite, from 1912, is of 'strikers dancing on a beach'[2] although in fact they are up to their ankles in water. They have their trousers rolled up to the knees; one wears braces. They are in an open embrace, facing front, as if they are dancing out of the past towards us. Elsewhere, others gather in the courtyard in the centre of a *conventillo*, one of the tenement buildings where whole families lived crowded into one room.

As it developed, the dance was learned by closely watching those who had become masters of the art. A novice would attend the men-only *práctica* for an 'apprenticeship' of up to three years, observing and then learning as a 'follower' – that is, to dance what was traditionally seen as the woman's role. Only when the learning was deemed to be secure would the new recruit graduate to the milonga and be allowed to dance with a woman. (Some commentators have suggested that an approach that builds on understanding the woman's point of view before engaging is the very opposite of machismo.) There are old *milongueros* (literally 'men who frequent milongas', often used to signify traditional dancers) still seen in the dance halls of Buenos Aires – Osvaldo 'Honey Feet' Cartery,* for example – who learned this way. And some of the cool young dancers I have met in Argentina don't take lessons, either. Instead they dance as many nights as they can afford, studying the experts, working creatively with a partner, developing and practising what works best with the music.

In the early 1900s, the music evolved hand in hand with the dance, the players amateurs, their music improvised. Now some of the earliest tangos survive only due to the efforts of groups such as the Orquesta Típica Sans Souci patiently transcribing old recordings. The first ensembles were probably trios, but by 1920 the norm for the tango band was the sextet: two violins, piano, double bass plus two of the instrument that, more than any other, has come to represent the sound and soul of tango: the bandoneon. A type of concertina produced almost exclusively in Germany, the bandoneon was named after its inventor Heinrich Band. Envisaged as a portable organ, it was intended originally for religious use. The bandoneon is notoriously difficult to play, with seventy-one buttons arranged in two sets on either side of the central bellows.

By the first quarter of the twentieth century, expert *bandoneonistas* were among the professional musicians

---

* This was true at the time of writing. Sadly, Osvaldo Cartery died in 2015.

beginning to be attracted to tango. Some travelled to Europe, where there were better opportunities for recording. The orchestras grew in size and variety. Although tango retained its foothold in the outer *barrios* and the improvised dance halls in the poorer south of Buenos Aires, orchestras such as that led by pianist and composer Carlos di Sarli gravitated to the wealthier north, where they became known for smooth and elegant playing. Much of the music prized by today's tango dancers comprises the tunes of 'the Golden Age' of tango, the sweet or mournful melodies of the 1930s and 40s – rather than Hollywood versions of tango or the moody strains of the Gotan Project, familiar from film, television and advertising.

Although tango in Argentina was essentially an urban, working-class phenomenon, its arrival in Europe in the first decades of the twentieth century (courtesy of the sons of the wealthiest Argentinians travelling to Paris to study or as part of their grand tour) saw its transformation into a chic pursuit for the middle and upper classes, and then into a fever that swept through the northern hemisphere. Its influence was reflected in developments in fashion – both in fabrics and in colours. Unlike the Charleston, which demanded above-the-knee skirts, tango created a vogue for long dresses with slits that allowed dancers to perform the long strides and dips required without revealing the moves of the dance itself. Elaborate headdresses also became associated with the dance.[3]

In Argentina, by the 1920s the phenomenon that had once been the preserve of the poor had become popular in more respectable circles. Dance venues and cabarets proliferated, and the period saw the establishment of many of today's best-loved orchestras. The peak of its popularity came in 1940. Orchestras were in such demand that they had to be hired a year in advance and newspapers carried pages of advertisements for dances.[4]

The 1950s saw the start of a thirty-year period of political and economic upheaval for Argentina, with inevitable repercussions in the world of tango. A series of military coups created a climate of fear and repression where expression of nationalistic feeling was discouraged and meetings of more than three people were banned. Many tango artists were imprisoned or blacklisted, and the demand for tango orchestras withered. One or two milongas survived but were hidden away.

In contrast, the arrival of rock and roll from the United States was encouraged by the government. An Argentinian friend of mine, Elisa, remembers the excitement of this new craze, which saw young people – herself and her friends included – jiving in the aisles in cinemas and concert halls. For Elisa then, tango was a dance for old people. It was not until the 1980s, with the collapse of the military regime and the emergence of touring shows, such as *Tango Argentino*, that the regeneration began. Now you can go to any city in the developed world and, maybe down a back street or in a church hall or above a café, you will hear the unmistakable sounds of a tango from the Golden Age.

Tango teacher and dancer Santiago León reminds us that what many of us think of as a dance is in fact a three-part entity, the words to the songs joining music and dance to complete the trio. Non-Spanish speakers thus miss a key dimension, although it is not hard to become familiar with some of the more common motifs: *corazón* (the heart), not surprisingly, but also *la noche* (the night), *barrio* (neighbourhood), *la vida* (life), *la muerte* (death), *soledad* (loneliness), *oblivión* (oblivion) and, of course, *amor* (love). I have friends who don't speak Spanish* but who learn the lyrics of a song to help them understand the music, although the inclusion of Lunfardo, a Buenos Aires slang, can make it even trickier to unravel the meaning. Author Robert Farris Thompson remarks on the way we are nonetheless drawn to 'decode' the texts, and the thrill of the process:

> They make you realise that there is this wondrous city far to the south, where the brave and the gifted are battling for love and for livelihood ... They write us reports from the front.[5]

Even if the sense of these postcards from the battleground eludes us at times – we struggled to find a convincing translation for the title of Osvaldo Pugliese's lovely recording of 'Farol' ('Lamp Post'),[†] for example – the subject matter

---

* The language is often referred to in Argentina as *Castellano*.
† Lyrics by Homero Expósito.

of tango is itself a shared language; food for the hungry, solidarity in difficulty.

But this thematic common ground does not always extend to matters of etiquette. One of the conventions that can offend those new to tango is its apparently inflexible male–female roles. My fiercely independent friend, Ginny, had visibly to grit her teeth through three hours of following the lead of a man in her first lesson (actually her only class; she never came back). To those familiar with the tango world, things are less clear. From the first moments of the embrace, 'leader' and 'follower' enter a dialogue, a relationship that lasts as long as the song. Each partner aims for absolute presence, total attention to the other, and trust – in each other, in the self, in the relationship. Yes, the man steers the journey of the couple, and in this sense the most useful thing the follower can do is wait, but this voluntary and temporary surrender is in itself a statement of faith. *I have confidence in you and in your ability to lead us through these moments*, the woman is saying. *But I also trust you to listen to me, even if I respond in a way that you do not expect.* As in any conversation, the leader's next move must stem from this response, rather than what he had hoped his partner would say. Two provisos: firstly, it is the follower's responsibility to be active in the dance, to contribute fully to the conversation; a passive follower will be able to do little more than follow; and secondly, despite the views of some who object, there are no rules that prevent a woman leading another woman – or indeed, remembering those early photographs, two men dancing together. In my experience, there is a different dynamic dancing with a female leader, and I have seen wonderful examples of the shared lead in a male–male couple.

As March drew to a close and the day of my departure to Argentina approached, I veered between excitement and trepidation. Would my courage hold? Would I discover that the private lessons, the group classes and the milongas had been enough to build my confidence and competence, or would I encounter a repeat of the terrors of my first two visits to the country? In a few days I would know, and it mattered so much. Tango is a lifestyle choice, at least for those of us who can travel with relative ease. But even for us, it is never going to be just a hobby. In one of those pointless arguments with a non-dancing friend, I found myself attempting to defend tango's unique qualities, particularly in relation to someone with Parkinson's. 'It could be anything,' Mart said. 'Darts, or Cumberland wrestling, or anything – whatever floats your boat. Anything that makes you feel better, takes you out of yourself, gets you meeting other people.' No. Even if you could add together the best of these pastimes with the key benefits offered by, say, ballet, bowling and embroidery, it would not approach the power of Argentine tango.

It is possible, I suppose, for a European like me to make the dance a kind of regular nibble at the exotic and leave it there, rather like the well-to-do Parisians of the 1920s. However, on earlier trips to Buenos Aires, once we got past the tango for tourists, what we found seemed closer to its working-class roots, danced by people who had made their living in the dance halls of the capital for fifty years, or who still went from work to tango and back to work with hardly a nod at the pillow. Absolutely an art form in its own right, it was also part of ordinary life, a necessary escape from reality in a country when reality was often hard to stomach; tango was not always particularly smart or glamorous, but it was in the blood. Worryingly, while tourism had helped to ensure the future of tango, I wondered if it was beginning to threaten ease of access for those who needed it most? I didn't know what the cost of entry to milongas would be now – the last time I was there, the price had trebled since my first visit. And this wasn't only an unselfish worry. The sustenance I gained from tango didn't derive from the package produced for visitor or for export; it needed to be the real thing. I had an image of a hand stretching out across the world to offer me, incredibly, 'the sense of being completely known, completely understood and completely accepted'.[6] What other 'hobby' could offer me that?

Lesson notes

One thing I'm sure about is that I have to have her trust.

— *John*

We are working on preparation for a step. 'You are reaching back,' John says, 'but I need to feel you preparing sooner; not moving, not reaching back, but being ready. I need to feel you are there for me, supporting me, supporting my step.' We move to the practice hold, watching my feet. 'Being ready' seems to involve moving my weight onto what becomes my standing leg and engaging the muscles in the free leg and along the side of the ribcage right up to the armpits – where, in tango theory, the legs begin. The free leg is poised, the foot resting on the floor but bearing no weight, ready to move but also relaxed so that, as I push off with the standing leg, bending the knee (do I?), it moves freely into the step. This may seem obvious to some, but it's new to me. I had believed myself ready and moving promptly, but there is a sense John has to wait for me to catch up.

Back in close embrace, we practise. Is that right? Is this what you mean? Can you see my feet in the mirror? 'I don't need to see your feet. I can feel... Yes.' Soon he is satisfied, and we move on. There is a bit of a pattern here: does it simply take a while for me to warm up? Or is this somehow a feature of the condition – that a response will need to be kick-started every time, the damaged brain tricked into a pre-damage state?

Now, focusing on 'more active' feet, we move on to back *ochos*. 'Go on,' he says, several times. 'Go on, then.' I go, eventually. I must seem reluctant. In fact, the lead is subtle, and either I have missed it or recognised it too late. 'I think you don't want to go there and end up doing something else instead.' We practise. 'I need you to twist more. Your upper body needs to stay with me, not go away from me. How much twist do you have?' We compare turning from the waist, first to one side, then the other. There is little difference between us. We practise. 'The walking is good, now. It's great. I could walk like this all day and not feel tired.' We squeeze in one last dance. As I put my shoes on, I try again to explain about confidence: how a follower may fear a telling-off if she gets it wrong. I give an example from this week's milonga. 'He had no right to speak to you like that,' John says. Time for the train. I'm excited, frustrated, disappointed, determined and energised. Good old dopamine, zinging round my nervous system, handing off the tiredness from the workout and the routine exhaustions of the day. Now, home to pack my tango shoes and my Buenos Aires bus timetable – and then off to the other side of the world.

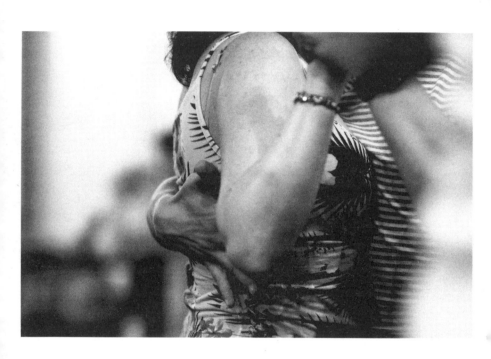

April:
Postcards

Buenos Aires, Tuesday 5th
Late nights. Street life. Tango.

I blame Francesca: when we staggered in at 3 a.m., her idea of a *boina por la noche* (literally a nightcap) had us opening an eight-peso bottle of red, so another four o'clock bedtime. Fine if you can sleep until noon, but the lure of the early mornings is irresistible – warm sun in an amazingly blue sky, the smell of coffee and that seductive auditory mix: dogs squalling, laughter, the screech and roar of traffic – someone leans a hand on a horn, three notes on an electric guitar from a nearby building, and from the little courtyard beyond the bathroom window, an acoustic guitar strummed. This morning, the clop of hooves: two men on the back of a cart, one (astride a battered white tank) shouting for business like a rag-and-bone man: is it ice he's selling? In the ventilation shaft, the sound of pigeons having sex. So Nancy says.

We are in San Telmo, a crumbling *barrio* within walking

distance of the wide avenues (the trees!) and towering buildings of the centre. Its history, the history of the city in miniature, is reflected in the muddle of nineteenth-century grandeur and concrete grot. I'm sharing a second-floor apartment with Nancy and John (another John), and Francesca; fellow Cumbrians Maggi and Pip and Alan and Claire are staying round the corner. From here, high ceilings and tall, shuttered and balconied windows look onto the narrow street. Everywhere a bombardment of sensation: a biblical storm; rain bouncing in the headlights of stalled taxis; walking along Libertad, block after block of jewellers. En route to shoe shopping, we come upon what might have been a scene from a film: a young man, well dressed, suddenly appears round the corner ahead of us, sprinting past at a tilt and carrying what looks like a tray of food for lunch. A straggle of ten or twelve pursuers bursts round the corner after him, jaws set, arms pumping. A small crowd of observers collects.

And then there's tango. We have danced in the jolly crowd at Leonesa, under the stars (and under lightning and thunder, augmented by West African *candombe* drummers) in Plaza Dorrego, in the friendly (if rather elderly) warmth of El Arranque and in the perennial favourite, Club Gricel – last night both hectic and welcoming. There are few tourists, though we get a strong sense of the melting pot that is this wonderful part of the world. Last night's partners included a twirling chap from Patagonia, a resident of Peru who came originally from Cornwall, several *porteños* (natives of the port, so locals), Ricardo 'El Turco' from Lebanon, and a genial gent who pronounced my tentative efforts 'unforgettable'. As we sat on in Gricel (there are plenty of examples on YouTube), an old charmer paused at our table, smiled and planted one of those audible kisses on my cheek, murmuring, *'Hola, buenas noches, qué tal?'* as he passed. Did he mistake me for someone else? Or am I becoming a recognisable part of the tango family?

Tigre Delta/Buenos Aires, Friday 15th
Tigre Delta. Culture Shock. Tango. Espanish.

The 'Tigre Delta Tour' for my birthday. We became proper tourists for the day, driven out through the opulence and – as Laura the tour guide put it – 'acquisitive power' of the northern suburbs to Tigre, a town on an island in the lower part of the Paraná Delta, a vast area of over 5,000 channels. The water is brown; not pollution, Laura told us, but a sediment of sand, clay and mud that settles as the waters of the river slow, to form constantly growing and shifting islands. As well as holiday accommodation, these islands supply the plywood and paper industries, and osiers are grown for wickerwork. There are no roads, cars or bridges. The only transport and all services (supermarkets, rubbish collection, medical support) are delivered by boat. With our *capitán* (what was his name?) and Ezekiel, our 'sailor', we daydreamed our way past a magical world of backwaters and reed beds, dilapidated landing stages and half-hidden houses on stilts, each looking for the perfect setting, imagining a different life.

Most of the time, however, we avoid tourist hotspots and soak up the experience of a different culture. At every corner there are contrasts and contradictions. Half a block from a state-of-the-art lighting shop, a figure sleeps beneath a sheet under a flyover. The return from Tigre took us in minutes from the leafy avenues of Belgrano and Olivos past the notorious Villa 31, a shantytown housing some 120,000 inhabitants, many of them illegal immigrants, in a clutter of corrugated iron, cardboard and rubble. On the way to collect our free tickets for the opera (the government's commitment to the arts is reflected in its spending: massive free concerts on the main highway by the Obelisco monument are commonplace – we missed Placido Domingo by a whisker), Tom Jones sings 'Sex Bomb' on the taxi radio. We walk miles of broken pavements, dodging spilling rubbish and exhaust-billowing buses, squeeze onto packed trains in the Subte metro, where scissor-sellers and entertainers (Janie saw a magic show) are treated with courtesy and generosity. We have a lesson in the *chacarera*, the folkloric dance that interrupts every milonga, hitching up our skirts and clicking our fingers obediently. We pick our way through skateboarders and step-sitters and kids in school uniform to one of the biggest modern art galleries in South America, just down the street. A man sits on the knobbly base of a tree at the end of our block, writing in a notebook, a dictionary on his knee.

Even tango is something of a culture shock, in the best possible way. Tonight we won't start until eleven, at a milonga out of town somewhere; a family occasion, some food, no doubt a demo. Last night we went out to the suburbs to a *práctica* (mixed, now – the days of men-only practices long gone) in a garage, where we had a wonderful *milonga traspié* lesson the previous week at the hands of experts Rino and Haydee. We were welcomed, of course, as if we were family. The verdict? As much fun as you can have with your clothes on. We have tended towards the traditional milongas: old school, few tourists, mainly older dancers (some have danced more or less every night for forty or fifty years). Occasionally, there are youngsters – early or mid-teens perhaps, smart-suited, hair slicked, the *milongueros* of the future? There is a vogue for the painted lady – the older woman whose face is completely obscured by make-up and botox – which we find disquieting. Prized venues often combine plain, glossed walls and a bit of plaster ceiling-decoration with tablecloths and hard chairs. The floor is everything. In La Nacional, a single row of men seated along one side regards the line of *chicas* opposite, an echo of the school dance: we watch for the *cabeceo*, that moment of eye contact, the hint of a nod, which signals an invitation to dance. Now, those who approach our table and ask – or, worse, point – seem rude. The world of the club is more familiar: the stylish Porteño y Bailarín, or the young and beautiful at Maldita, where the excellent Orquesta Típica El Afronte play live on Wednesdays.

The vagaries of language continue to baffle and delight, and there is always a question. *'Una pregunta: hay cambio?'* because there never is any change. 'Is there a lady in the toilet?' has become our code for, 'Do I need a couple of pesos for a tip?' 'How was that dance?' 'It was "absolutely nice",' (to quote Francesca's new friend Alejandro). Who amongst us has the strongest claim as founder member of the 'English Rowing Club' ('rowing' rhyming with 'ploughing', in Laura's lexicon)? The two married couples fought over the privilege. And everybody's favourite – from Francesca, of course – as we looked up at the third-floor balcony sign *Mónica Fux: Estudio de Danzas*: 'I wonder what she does for a living?'

Buenos Aires, Tuesday 26th
Music and movement. Win some, lose some. The perfect tango.

On Friday night we squeeze into a combi, which takes us out to Flores for Milonga La Baldosa. Despite its marble floors, the venue is local and familial rather than glamorous, (though the hip and famous and delicious dancers slid in, and onto the dance floor, as we were leaving, at around 2:30 a.m.). An impressive and endearing demonstration from Gustavo Chaile and Ayelen Morando (aged sixteen and fifteen!) and the wonderful Orquesta Típica Sans Souci with singer Chino Laborde – theatrical, humorous, posturing, a cross between an Irish poet and a taller version of Welsh writer Dylan Thomas. A proper jobbing band, they played from transcriptions of rare live recordings of the orchestra of bandoneonist and composer Miguel Caló, their music untidy, photocopied sheets of what looked like handwritten staves and notes, which occasionally flew off their stands. The old bandoneon maestro in the centre grinned encouragement at his young neighbour as they delivered familiar tunes with the extra sweetness of a live performance. Such a contrast despite the similar line-up (violins, double bass, three or four bandoneons, piano and singer) with the funky, passionate edge of El Afronte.

As we danced our way round the different milongas, I began to recognise characteristic features of orchestras already half familiar from recordings I'd danced to in the UK – Biagi, and Donato and De Angelis. I experienced the delights of the late-Pugliese *tanda*. I relished the exotic medley of sounds: *candombe* drummers on Defensa on a Sunday evening, mobbed by a pavement crowd that can't keep still, then sounds of a practice behind a closed door into the night, the title track of Beirut's album *The Flying Club Cup* the anthem of choice in San Telmo's boutiques and restaurants, the plastic-panpipe trill of what we think must be an itinerant knife-grinder (not the postie, as we believed originally), guitar echoing up the stairwell or a few chords from the street-corner boys, the mournful sounds of Hugo Díaz's harmonica . . .

I danced the last of a *tanda* with Alejandro, to his favourite 'Niebla del Riachuelo'. We spent an emotional afternoon in Plaza Dorrego, our reminiscences of our first steps interrupted by a recording of the Greek tango – which we danced to all those years ago with Raymond – then Esteban Morgado's version of 'Every Breath You Take', evoking memories of the gay milonga in 2008 where we watched a shared lead for the first time.

Win some, lose some. Losses: 1 forgotten bag (before we even got on the plane), 1 twelve-hour delay, 2 wallets & contents (stolen on the Subte), 1 septic toe (recovered not removed), 1 case of fluid on the knee, 1 mystery illness (cough/throat/fever/sunstroke), 1 eye infection, 1 lost false nail, all the ATMs out of cash on Mondays, 1 fractured heart . . . Wins: 1 shoe bag (with shoes) returned from the back of a taxi via a second taxi that gave chase, several late-night drivers who wait until we're safely back inside before driving off, many compliments on our dancing, numerous charming waiters, another rip-roaring *práctica* in Rino's garage, a date for Francesca tomorrow night with a bank-queue sleaze, a few Alejandros, a lovely apartment, wine/Quilmes beer/empanadas/wine/lunches, time spent with our Cumbrian tango teacher Lili and her mum Lidia, milongas/roof terraces/city streets/new shoes/skirts/sunshine/more wine. And Pip's wallet (plus all contents except the money) returned by a character called Alberto. And the cost? Having to listen to his apparently endless stream of stories – about his family, Sean Connery, the Red Cross – and the 100-peso tip that Pip gave him.

And the perfect tango? We argue endlessly about the 'feel', the embrace, what makes a good dancer, a muscular lead versus a subtle one, dancing on the music, how to be *floja* – the rag-doll-relaxed that Rino and his boys prize, how to recognise the face that goes with the shirt; the connection. We learn to avoid the gropers and the crashers and the spine-dislocators, each searching the other end of the world for someone with whom we can be totally in tune, who will meet our obsession equally, whole-heartedly. Occasionally, amongst all the fancy footwork and the twirling bodies, we glimpse a moment of mutual delight as two faces revolve in front of us with the same smile, or we hold our breath as a couple remains poised, motionless for long seconds, before easing into synchronous movement. If we are lucky, we experience one or two such moments ourselves. And the shredded toes, swollen ankles, scraped shins and tears – what Claire calls our 'disasters'? On balance more heaven than hell, but the Louise Bourgeois exhibition we visit provided an answer of sorts, on a handkerchief embroidered by the artist (1996):

I HAVE BEEN
TO HELL AND
BACK.
AND LET ME
TELL YOU,
IT WAS WONDERFUL.[1]

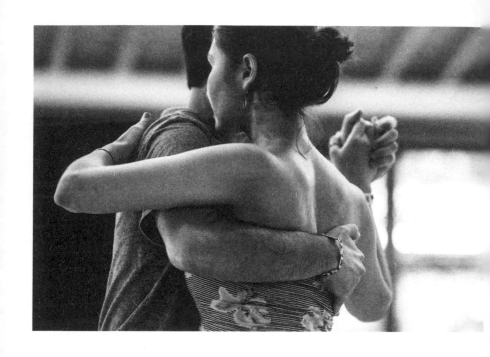

May:
Grace and Favour

So what is it about tango that has the power to transform?
Sceptics often add a second question: 'Is it just…?' Answer:
No, it's not 'just'… the rhythm, or the music, or any one
aspect which makes tango different from aerobics or
cycling, or even salsa or ballroom. I've read much of the
research material that describes and records the impact
tango seems to have on an individual with Parkinson's, and
in some cases speculates about why and how this works.
In my own experience, each feature of the dance hits a
particular Parkinson's spot, with dramatic results.

Take the element of grace. I'm no football fan, but
watching a talented player control a ball for ten or twelve
paces is infinitely satisfying: that combination of timing,
poise, agility, fluency, dodge and weave, halt and go –
wonderful, especially as these are skills I will never share.
The grace of the *tanguero* is akin to that of the practised
midfielder, and I am not just talking about professional
dancers. Of course, we also enjoy these qualities in

performances, along with the complex motifs and patterns that ordinary mortals will never match. But what often draws that gasp of delight from those watching is a quieter, more private moment – perhaps a hiatus before a step, or a second or two where the balance of the follower is deliberately upset and then restored. Moments such as these are the stuff of the milonga. On any evening, almost every couple will touch on perfection, that instant where everything comes together in the best possible way. And when you're not on the floor yourself, look around: at every turn – amongst the clumsy and overambitious, fat or thin, skippers or gliders, shufflers or stalkers – the surprise of beauty.

Off the dance floor, those with Parkinson's rarely achieve grace. It is common both to become 'stuck', unable to move when you wish, and to be unable to be still when you choose, beset by tremors and twitches which rattle on in spite of your best efforts to stop them. Characteristic movement aberrations include unpredictable stopping and starting, or moments spent teetering on the brink of motion followed by a sudden lunge. (A friend of mine, who also has Parkinson's, walks with a frame. When we last met, I watched as he visibly prepared himself, hesitating as though there was a large obstacle in his path, before setting off across the floor in a high-energy, high-velocity shuffle.) Balance, too, is notoriously problematic. Tango presents a challenge to any dancer. For those with Parkinson's, the challenge is doubled; but then, so, perhaps, is the benefit.

You could say that grace begins with posture. The correct posture is so fundamental to tango, and so tricky to get right, that many classes, even for advanced dancers, begin with attention to this area. Different teachers have different ways of describing what is required: upright is often how it begins, head up, chin tucked in slightly, spine straight, shoulders relaxed. This in itself was a challenge for me. After years of struggle with posture, I found myself tending towards textbook signs of parkinsonism: a stoop, a poked-out head, a middle fold, a slumping chest. Or, now that I was in my sixties, were these merely signs of growing older? Certainly there were times when extreme fatigue made it feel impossible to hold myself upright. And I'm sure there were psychological issues, too. The emotional toll[1] of the condition is well documented. When I was feeling low, or especially unattractive or clumsy, I tended to retreat into a kind of defensive isolation, a closing-in. Standing tall, head up, chest open, was the last thing I felt like doing. If you are serious about tango, though, this is what you have to do.

You may be asked to start with a rocking motion, forward and back, side to side, shifting the weight from the heel to the ball of the foot, from one foot to another, from the outside to the inside of the foot, and then to find your centre. The notion of a central axis is crucial: the analogy of a thread running up from the feet to the crown of the head is often used. I like the metaphor of a conduit, a channel that needs to be kept open, unobstructed by kinks or compressions that will interrupt the flow. By extension, this image is also good for staying in your axis: if the channel slips off centre, not only will the liquid not flow freely, but the whole structure will topple. Again this targets a key facet of the Parkinson's experience: balance. Long before diagnosis, I was aware of insecurities here, a tendency to wobble when it was most inconvenient (on a northern hillside, for example). Does this mean I had a predisposition to Parkinson's? Or that, as some suspect, the line between disease and health is less definite than we imagine? One piece of genome research found 'striking similarities' between healthy ageing brains and the brains of people with diseases such as Alzheimer's.[2] What was clear was that, although the disease had undoubtedly progressed, my ability to remain in my axis on the dance floor had increased dramatically in the first few months of the year and the improvements had been sustained – or had sustained me – on dance floors on the other side of the world.

Of course, some support is derived from the partner: while we may each practise alone, we dance as a couple. Still, the deal is that you are responsible for your own axis. It is not acceptable to hang on to your partner, to pull on them or expect them to hold you up. This means you have to get your core working for you, using and developing muscles that may have given up expecting calls to action from the damaged brain. These muscles must carry on working for you as you dance, in order to maintain that critical connection with your partner. Like a martial art, tango demands core strength and control. While muscle damage does not necessarily follow from Parkinson's, mood and confidence may well have rendered these areas lazy, at least. To take on tango could be a wake-up call.

Your other 'friend' – to borrow a favourite image from those who have taken part in workshops led by Netherlands-based teacher Eric Jeurissen – is the floor. The idea of working with the floor, consciously feeling it as each foot lands, is a useful notion for those whose balance is compromised.

Back on home turf, the complexities of posture entered my awareness every time I picked up my tango shoe bag. (There is a school of thought that recommends that Parkinson's dancers should avoid heels. Isn't that like recommending paper aeroplanes for pilots? I might have just passed on my highest black-and-silver beauties but, while I wobbled at times, on the dance floor I was rarely troubled by real instability or fear of falling in the same way that I was out in the wider world.) Struggling to fasten the straps of my shoes, I would prepare to stretch and unfurl my aching back as I rose to my feet, wary of those uncertain moments before I found my centre. Searching for a sense of the perfect tension between up and down, feeling the firmness of the floor as I stood tall, I would recall the group lesson that had used a tai chi motif to highlight the dual energy required – one hand palm upwards, pushing up, the other palm facing downwards and pushing down, as we walked. The delicate balance between these two directions is beautifully illustrated in Simon Armitage's poem 'Mother, Any Distance',[3] where the critical steadiness of the anchor contrasts with the freedom of a kite: the dancer needs to be grounded but at the same time free to fly. As I walked onto the floor and prepared to meet my partner, I kept these up-and-down energies in mind, and listened, not just to the music: I listened with my body for my partner's intention, beginning that process of negotiation – of finding the best arrangement, the strongest connection with that person in that moment – even if this was someone I had danced with many times before. Almost past the thinking stage, I would strive to be 100 per cent present, as though every muscle, every nerve ending, every atom of myself was focused on this instant, actively engaged in communication with this other. And as the music took hold, the process of transformation would begin.

As I eased myself back into Cambridge's tango community, it was clear that the support I gained from regular private lessons, originally intended specifically to prepare for Argentina, was too precious to give up while the funds, and John's patience, lasted. Looking back, I suppose at the simplest level the lessons offered a radical alternative to the feelings of failure that come with Parkinson's territory. For an hour, I was special, not in spite of the condition but in part because of it – refusing to be held back by its disabling aspects, working at the complexities of the dance alongside an expert. I thought of the ladders in Joan Miró's paintings[4]: as well as an escape from the tricky realities of the rest of life, tango was, like Miró's ladders, an opportunity to aim for the stars. I think it was Picasso who said that art 'washes away from the soul the dust of everyday life'. To have gone from my own small repertoire of movement disorders to the possibility of grace, the art of Argentine tango and the transformations it was creating seemed little short of a miracle.

Lesson notes

As I walk up the path, the door is open. Electronic tango is playing – unusual – but changes to Francisco Canaro's 'Hotel Victoria' by the time I have my shoes on. I tell my Córdoba story: there to carry out research for my novel, Francesca and I trailed round the city looking for a place to stay one very crowded holiday weekend and came upon the hotel immortalised in the song. It even had vacancies, as we discovered when we enquired at the reception desk; they actually showed us an available room. Unfortunately, behind the romantically crumbling façade it was a building site, undergoing a major refurbishment that filled its grand interior with the din of machinery and brick dust.

I'm sure John has heard the story before but of course he's too polite to say so, and anyway these first few minutes are precious orientation time; focusing time, setting aside whatever we've turned up with and finding a middle ground, a way we can be together. The doors are open into the garden, the air cool between showers. I feel calm: for once I have slept well. I stand in front of the photos on the wall (family photos that I've looked at many times for their steadying effect) while he makes tea. I chase a bee back out into the garden. We dance. The door bangs repeatedly until he props it open with a stone. He doesn't like the Canaro today, changes it for De Angelis, apologises for being fidgety and adjusts the volume. And now it's time. We begin.

'So – *ochos*,' he says. He shows the small pivot needed for back *ochos* in the close embrace and we practise, keeping the pivot separate from the step but aiming for more fluidity. Then into the *molinete* – back *ocho*, side step, into the cross – or, in an open embrace, the pivot – before the return; don't rush the step. Is this right? It feels like an area I've been familiar with for a while but have been fudging slightly. John reminds me to let the pivot work its way up to my lower torso while maintaining attention to him in my upper body. I can practise this. 'These can be beautiful,' I think he says. Does he say this? And now into the *giro*: the full turn, right round, looking at the last steps. Beyond the open doors, the garden gets its next drenching, and the hiss and stipple of the tumbling rain overlays the music. A couple of waltzes. 'Lovely, very waltzy,' he says.

A mention of Pugliese brings the next change in music. We work out that the song 'Nochero Soy' must mean something like 'I am of the night' (simply 'nocturnal', I think later) and move on to 'La Rayuela' – 'tangle', I suggest, although this turns out to be wrong; in fact it means 'hopscotch'. The music insists on stretch and suspend, reach and hold, the large compass of the dance echoed in another colossal downpour. And then the distraction of meanings leads me to a forgotten discovery, that 'Sinsabor' (by Edgardo Donato's orchestra) means 'problem' or 'trouble', usually related to love. 'A wonderful song,' he says. 'It needs to be danced strongly.' And we do. Time for another? I talk about the difficulty of relaxing the upper body while trying to keep the lower half working. As we finish, all that rain leads me into the story – how many stories? It's a wonder I learn anything – of a family camping trip on the Isle of Arran, when we put the tent up in a deluge, almost coming to blows. The storm continued long into the night, but in the morning we woke to a world rinsed clean. The tide was out – miles of pale mud dotted with hundreds of rocks. Then one rock moved, and another: a bay full of seals, basking in the early-morning sun, their ends curled up like bananas.

On the train, my head rings with the sweet rhythms of the waltz. Although grace dissolves fast, I feel strong, coordinated and energised well into the afternoon. Almost six months in, the lessons have become an essential factor in my well-being, and I feel I am making progress, although muddles in the evening dances remind me of Lenin: one step forward, two steps back.

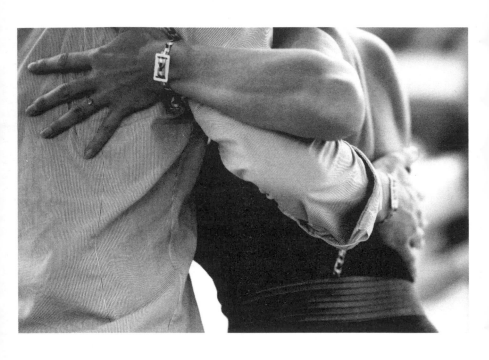

June:
Movement

*When I put on my leading shoes and look around the room,
I'm keen to dance with Kate. She is a mature dancer, with
years of practice, thought and consideration in her body, and
it shows. Kate gets the idea of true connection; she listens
intently for my lead. There is sometimes a slow heaviness
or delay in some of her movements, but as a consequence I
do not need to worry that Kate will predict, rushing ahead
on her own and leaving me behind. In fact, this possibly
contributes to her excellent presence. Dare I say it? Maybe
the P-word sometimes brings something positive to the dance.*

— *Ellie*

Two minor memories: the first, maybe ten years ago,
a regular Thursday-night practice in Carlisle's beautiful
fifteenth-century Tithe Barn. I am dancing with Raymond.
For the second or third time, as we approach the *barrida* –
that lovely moment where the leader sweeps the follower's
foot sideways with his own foot – I wobble, then freeze and

apologise. 'Don't worry, darling,' Raymond says, 'though I wonder what it is?' The second memory: three years later, a Monday evening, and Francesca and I have made the short trip over the border into Scotland. We are in Victoria Hall in Annan. I have paid John – another John – ten pounds, I think, for some consolidated practice before our next trip to Argentina. 'Well, OK,' he says, 'though there seems to be some sort of *delay*...'

Functional mobility – the range of movement needed for normal daily living – is compromised in Parkinson's. Bradykinesia, slow movement, is one of the less dramatic signs. It's uneven, unpredictable, intermittent, selective. It tends to be less of an issue during dedicated exercise – walking the Norfolk Coast Path with friends, for example, or heading on foot across London, from King's Cross to Trafalgar Square, I might be accused of doing a route march. But when getting to my feet from a café table, walking onto the dance floor or eating a plate of food, progress is often exasperatingly slow, both for myself and, I imagine, those around me. This is exacerbated when I am trying to do something else at the same time (eat dinner and continue a conversation).[1] Difficulty initiating or responding to movement is at the root of what John in Cambridge described in our early lessons as 'lazy feet' or, more colourfully, the 'can't be arsed' effect. The term made me smile for the way it poked fun at something that was certainly more a symptom than a lack of effort. Somehow, I had to override whatever it was that was stopping me moving, and just do it. A tall order on the street, this somehow became possible in tango. How did this work? First I felt the pressure of expectation: the music, the embrace, the intention of my partner – all calling for me not just to take the step but to prepare for it, shifting the weight, engaging the muscles, getting the free leg ready. Simultaneously, I think, and equally strong, was the sensation of support from the music, from my partner and, at milongas, from the other couples who were poised at the same instant, so that to do the hard thing became the easiest option. And given the multitasking that tango demands, there was never just one thing to master – yet it was as if asking the impossible was what made it work. And the focus on waking up those sluggish feet, a repeated feature of our early lessons, soon faded from view.

There are other specific gait difficulties associated with Parkinson's. As well as speed (or the lack of it), individuals may struggle with turning, walking backwards and stride length. One study I referred to earlier highlighted the importance of external cues in helping those with Parkinson's to achieve 'nearly normal speed and amplitude'. The writers suggested that particular features of tango – stepping over or tapping a partner's foot, for example, as well as the cross (where the follower's left ankle comes to rest crossed in front of the right, transferring the weight to the left leg) – are similar to exercises used to help counteract freezing and may serve as visual cues.[2] The frequent weight changes demanded in tango also mirror a strategy used in treatment to address freezing. Perhaps regular dancing was keeping this at bay in my case? Although stride length was not a major issue for me generally – I had not yet reached the shuffling stage – I had certainly developed a tendency to take shorter steps in the dance. While this may have been part laziness and part an accommodation to those crowded Buenos Aires dance floors, I'm sure that some of the adaptation stemmed from insecurities with balance, and some from a general lack of confidence – a reluctance to commit to a step in case it was 'wrong'. So over the next few weeks John and I worked on positive stepping, stretching out when the lead or the music demanded, until I reached a point where I could enjoy the opportunity for that longer backward step.

For a follower, the back step is the norm, and I think the way it is achieved is one factor which makes tango so beneficial for the Parkinson's dancer, where the uncertainties of balance and posture encourage a tendency to lean back and, at worst, to fall in that direction. The follower is aware of her posture, upright but leaning slightly toward the leader. At all times (there are occasional exceptions) she is responsible for her own axis, but she has the support of the embrace and the energy of the leader, whose own centre is in a kind of collaborative counterbalance to her own. When her leader prepares to step forward, he almost draws her towards him before stepping. He is saying, 'Come with me, let's go together,' which is reassuring. The transfer of weight from one leg to the other feels smooth and sure. If this goes according to plan, the sensation of falling back, unpleasant for both partners, is avoided. It doesn't always go according to plan because, like many of tango's apparently simple movements, it's harder than it looks. The pleasure is in working towards the achievement, the satisfaction when it feels perfect. And for a dancer with Parkinson's, it is both a recipe for success on the dance floor and a model for movement elsewhere; in this respect, then, a transferable skill.

The nature of the forward step in tango means that it, too, can benefit dancers with Parkinson's. While some styles and much show-tango favour stepping onto the ball of the foot, many prefer a step where the heel lands a nanosecond ahead, and this can help to correct the Parkinson's tendency to walk with a 'flat foot strike',[3] where the whole foot lands at once. I discovered that a conscious attempt at a positive forward step, where the heel arrived first, particularly when part of a turn, was better for balance and stride length as well as helping to create enough momentum for a successful pivot.

Pivoting, twisting and turning on the spot are all fundamental to Argentine tango and can be seen to target the difficulties with turning experienced by those with Parkinson's. The pivot in particular is an integral part of the *ocho*, the figure of eight that the follower completes in two steps across the front of, or around, the leader, while keeping her upper body turned towards her partner, maintaining the chest-to-chest connection. We practised the technique in group classes and in our individual lessons, but whenever the task was set, I felt my stomach muscles contract with anxiety. My body became a lumbering weight, a sackful of turnips that slipped and lurched inside my skin, pulling me off-centre, gluing me to the ground. For months, perhaps years, I managed without the pivot entirely when I could get away with it, substituting small steps for that ball-of-the-foot spin that looks so beautiful and so easy when executed by an expert. And as for 'disassociation', the ambitious mid-body twist that sends the hips and legs in one direction while holding the chest and shoulders steady – these aspects of the dance are complicated for the best of us. However, it repeatedly seemed as if it was precisely this sense of a step-too-far which took me towards a breakthrough. Perhaps this was partly due to physical contact with my partner's hands – even the lightest touch is known to help with postural stability.[4] But I was sure it was also a refusal to be defined by the condition, and an acceptance that continual challenge was crucial to my motor rehabilitation. Contrary to those who suggested that certain 'figures' or patterns of steps – the lovely *molinete*, for example, where the follower traces a circular grapevine pattern around the leader – 'may be too challenging to the stability of the average participant with PD',[5] I wanted it to be hard.

The biggest challenge of Argentine tango does not lie in the complexity of the steps, however. Unlike sequence dances, where couples work through a set routine, tango is improvised, with frequent changes in pace, rhythm and direction. Although there are figures which may be taught in classes and repeated in practice, they rarely occur in the dance predictably or in their entirety. They are, rather, the vocabulary that the dancers draw on to build their conversation. If the role of the leader is to initiate and guide this conversation in response to the music and to his partner, the follower's challenge is to listen, to be so much in tune with her partner's intention that she moves with him at his speed, in the direction he chooses, taking her time to maintain elegance without falling behind, matching his energy with her own. This is no easy matter. It requires full attention, stillness, balance, confidence and control of movement – any or all of which are likely to be problematic for someone with Parkinson's. The music supports the dancer, but also demands an active response, from the follower as well as the leader.

Many lovers of the dance are drawn to explore the music. It is an astonishingly rich resource: a hundred years of history spanning North America, South America, Europe and Scandinavia (did you know that Finland has its own thriving tango scene?), from full orchestras to solo harmonica, instrumental and voiced, contemporary urban or Golden Age, laughing rhythms or mournful evocations of loss. My tastes have changed as I've listened and learned more. Whatever the style or period, though, dancing to a favourite tango can feel as if the music is actively helping you to move fluently and gracefully. And perhaps it is. For once, it seems, something that often feels more like a guilty pleasure than anything else is good for you. And if you have Parkinson's, it is especially good for you.

Lesson notes

Friday's lesson was prefaced by a minor disaster, a result of house-hunting. I'd progressed from my brother's sofa to a tiny flat by the river, but the prospect of a tenant for my Cumbrian house as an unfurnished rental meant I had to find somewhere in Cambridge to accommodate all my furniture. I'd cycled along the river to Chesterton to view a disarmingly impractical Victorian cottage, all gangly hollyhocks, sprawling wisteria and draughty windows. Cycling back in the rain across the common, the bike wheels skewed sideways on a bend and I was on the ground. I made it to the train, aware of a sticky wet patch under the torn knee of my trousers, then spent ten minutes on a chair in the kitchen with cotton wool and hot water, John holding back the tiny flaps of skin on my knee while I dug out fragments of gravel. 'You can have the lesson another time,' he said. 'Now I think you need to get this into a hot bath.' No, I said, suddenly awash with an eleven-year-old's tears. I'm fine. I really want to stay. Don't make me go home.

We started with Canaro's ebullient rhythms (in 'Pampa') and then some D'Arienzo, with the predictable interruption while I explained the pronunciation of the double 'r' in 'El Entrerriano' (why do I never shut up?). Strangely, I felt capable and reasonably focused, able to respond quickly and dance on the beat: the adrenaline from the fall, perhaps, or the after-effects of the previous evening's milonga, where for once my body seemed ready to perform what was expected? One of the features of Parkinson's is its on–off nature, so that I am never sure whether things will work, or whether we will have that delay effect, all fuzzy head and leaden legs. This makes the pivot particularly tricky – I recognise exactly what is expected, but my body simply feels too heavy for my legs to move – so tango's close embrace is a refuge: back *ochos* can be negotiated without a pivot, *milonguero*-style.*

Last time, we agreed the benefits of working in a more open embrace. Today John suggested I try *ochos* independently, without support. A quick attempt showed how difficult this was for me (although this may be due to years of laziness, when I didn't practise what I had learned) and we spent some minutes on forward and backward *ochos* in the lightest of practice frames, with an emphasis on me taking responsibility for my own axis and balance. Then the mirror exercise: upper body and chest facing the mirror, hips and feet at ninety degrees; a sidestep towards the mirror followed by a 180-degree pivot, so that the lower body now faced the opposite direction, while keeping the torso in place. This was challenging on two counts: the ordinary physical challenge of disassociation (or was this

---

* A term coined in the tango renaissance of the 1990s to describe a style of dance which harked back to a simpler style danced in Buenos Aires in the 1950s, a reaction against complex choreographies which had crept into social dancing.

'counter-rotation'?), where the lower and upper halves of the body move in opposite directions; and, somewhere in the damaged brain, where new learning feels impossible and a kind of panicky resistance kicks in. Both are useful challenges. I struggled with the exercise but came away determined to work at it. I feel sure that making it complicated is a good way forward; asking just a bit more than can easily be achieved, in the context of teaching that responds creatively and intuitively to the needs of the moment (cotton wool and all), and firm and trusted support. We finished with John's story of another dancer's progress dogged by lack of confidence, and a couple of dances in the comfort of the close embrace.

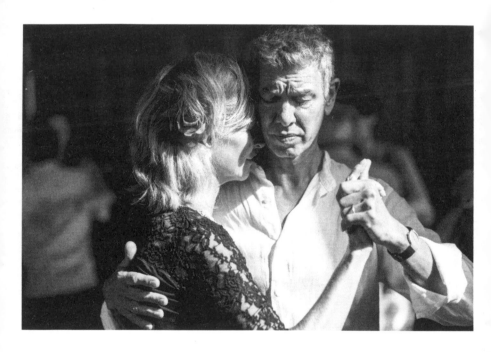

July:
Music

It seems to me that the tremors of Parkinson's can be suspended during movement, sometimes almost entirely for a whole tango. For a tango, or a number of tangos, Kate can move elegantly and get lost in the music with her partner, just like anyone else who has trained at this most difficult dance for several years. So I try to treat Kate not as a sufferer from Parkinson's but like anyone else who takes a class – listening to what she needs to attend to, encouraging gently towards a better quality of movement. It's an ongoing process, but so it is for all tango dancers, and the process can be enjoyable and rewarding.

— John

I have been thinking about music, about its place in my life, what I love, what I need. My earliest musical memory: singing 'Soldier, soldier, won't you marry me?', with actions, in North Road Primary School in Carnforth. Three or four years later: in the front room in Wembley, something loud and symphonic – Mahler, probably – my dad hectoring as he conducted. From about the same time: hours of piano practice punctuated by early Saturday-morning lessons in a house round the corner. I remember feeling sickened by the lingering smells of toast and sleep as the teacher brushed her long, yellow-grey hair. As I approached my teens, there were brief flirtations – Cliff's 'Living Doll', Carole King, Radio Luxembourg, the Sunday-afternoon charts – before a long, and sadly one-sided, love affair with Bob Dylan. When I was a student, I was introduced to opera, and saw The Who live before they became famous. I also met a choirmaster who claimed that he could liberate any young woman so that she could 'sing like a nightingale'. It didn't work for me. In fact, through forty years of enjoying listening to anything – from Bach to Bowie, folk to fusion – and five or six years playing the clarinet and saxophone, singing has continued to defeat me. My worst moment: Carlisle's annual Christmas pantomime in the Green Room Theatre on West Walls, one of my sixth-form students in the cast. He spots me in the audience and drags me up on stage. I stumble through the first verse (all of it) and chorus of 'I've Got a Lov-er-ly Bunch of Coconuts'. My son, Jack, almost a young man, is sitting in the front row of the audience, his face in his hands, sliding down in his seat as if he wants the ground to swallow him. In the secret places of my heart, though, I sing beautifully, and I feel that music runs through my arteries, lurking in muscle and bone marrow. Now, more than ever, it feels essential to my well-being. A friend with Parkinson's describes music as her food. I know what she means.

Revisiting Oliver Sacks' wonderful *Musicophilia* recently, I was reminded of the shock of recognition that accompanied my first reading. Between customers during my weekly stint in the local Amnesty bookshop, I had picked up the heavy hardback lying on the counter and turned straight to the chapter entitled 'Kinetic Melody: Parkinson's Disease and Music Therapy'.[1] Not only did I find an accurate description of the condition as turning the natural flow of movement into a 'kinetic stutter', but also an echo of words I myself had found to describe what had happened to me: 'graceless' was the term used by one patient quoted in the book. Writing of his work at New York's Beth Abraham Hospital in the 1960s, Sacks includes vivid depictions of the 'abyss' of parkinsonism, its 'flat, frozen landscape' offset against the extraordinary effects where music was present, when its tempo and speed proved more powerful than the condition and allowed patients to return to their 'own rate of moving'. The strongest resonance for me was Sacks' discovery of the power of music to 'awaken', not just to movement but to 'vivid emotions and memories, fantasies, whole identities'; in short, 'everything that L-dopa [a drug now widely used to treat Parkinson's], still in the future, was subsequently to do'. More than fifty years later, on a dance floor in Cambridge, I described to a friend what felt like a chemical rush as the music began. At the end of the evening, awash with the residue, sleep would elude me. With an established milonga habit and obsessive listening at home, regular injections of 'auditory dopamine' meant that a good night's sleep was becoming a rarity.

And, of course, it's not just any old music. I recall a between-dances chat where a partner said, 'Well, in tango there are only so many tunes, aren't there?' What?! I'm sure even the most practised tango DJ regularly discovers new possibilities. There are the lovely, melancholic Greek melodies; original compositions and adaptations from the group ZUM; reworked versions of old favourites by orchestras such as Color Tango; something sweet and husky sung in French; one-off delights from Tom Waits and Kristina Olsen; and all this in addition to the wealth and variety of tangos from the Golden Age.

Musically, tango is complex, rhythmically and melodically, although generalisations beyond this are probably no more helpful than blanket descriptions of jazz. Still, there are facets of the music that seem to impact directly on the symptoms of Parkinson's. Take the disease's rigidity, for example, that unrelenting stiffness which makes movement sluggish and sometimes painful, or the tendency to 'freeze'. A beautiful and lyrical slow piece, such as Francisco Canaro's 1935 recording of 'Poema', seems to ease tension and restore fluency. Sometimes it was played in the group classes as we worked on technique and I felt the tightness in my neck and shoulder muscles melt away at the first sweet and plaintive notes from the violin. When I discover that Canaro began his life in extreme poverty, started work at the age of ten as a shoeshine boy, spent his adolescence working in a factory and made his first violin out of wood and tin, I feel humbled. Still, by the end of successful career as an orchestra leader, performer and a prolific composer, he had travelled widely (he made his first visit to Paris in 1925), published his memoirs and had around 4,000 recordings to his name. In fact Canaro's is the only Golden Age recording of 'Poema' and there is famously a dark side to the song's story. Reputedly written on a train during a band tour of Germany by Mario Melfi and Eduardo Bianco, the lyrics contain a thinly veiled confession of Bianco's murder of his wife's lover.[2] Perhaps this helps to explain the intensity of feeling that the song carries?

For me, the emotional strength of tango's music lies at the heart of its power to transform, and this became a natural focus of my individual sessions with John. I recall one lesson which began with Osvaldo Fresedo's orchestra and their interpretation of the popular 'Niebla del Riachuelo' recorded in 1937. Roberto Ray is the singer, although technically, I learned years later, he is an *estribillista*, a singer of refrains, which explains why the voice enters late in the song, for just one chorus. In the 1930s and early 1940s, dance orchestras played mainly instrumental numbers; if there was a singer at all, he would sing just part of the lyrics. Ray's voice has a wonderful, almost-out-of-range tone that suggests it might crack with the weight of nostalgia as he repeats the title of the song, 'Niebla del Riachuelo'. *Niebla* is fog and the word *riachuelo* means 'little river' or 'creek', but in this song it refers also to a particular river on the southern edge of Buenos Aires. The Riachuelo, also known as the Matanza River, flows into the Rio de la Plata near La Boca, the 'mouth' of the river giving its name to the *barrio* most strongly associated with tango, due to the arrival of new immigrants who disembarked there.

The piece is a lament, the pain of loss emphasised in the insistent *nunca mas* (never again), perhaps reflecting the feelings of those who rushed to Europe in the 1920s under the spell of 'tangomania' and found themselves missing the city they had left behind. The song has a haunted quality, and those familiar with other versions will hear the ghostly echo of the lyrics omitted here – of the castaways and sunken ships, the coal tugs, the shadows and the bridges where the wind howls. At the same time, it is a love song – like many tangos, a song of love lost – and there is a lighter undercurrent in the rippling piano – or is it a harp? Elegiac rather than operatic, the song nonetheless reminds me of the closing moments of *La Traviata*, where the sadness of the action is transcended by the sweetness of the music. Or is it simply a sentimental evocation of a much-loved neighbourhood, an Argentinian 'Fog on the Tyne'?

As we danced, I heard the sounds of the water, the muted clank of machinery. I thought of the shanty town that has grown up along the Riachuelo's banks and found myself remembering that I had danced to the same tune with Alejandro in Club Maldita, San Telmo, just a few months before. For Alejandro, the song carried powerful personal memories and was the piece he associated with the birth of his love of tango. In an instant the mournful rhythms transported me back to the other side of the world, and we had to stop for tea and tissues.

There are more fulsomely melancholy tangos that reflect the displacement and alienation of those early immigrants and that speak to the search for what is lost or broken in all of us: 'Volver', 'Vuelvo al Sur', 'Nada' and so on. Perhaps these are part and parcel of a culture famous for its fondness for analysis, a desire to stay with and explore the pain rather than just cheer up. This seems to me more helpful than the approach of some 'tango therapists', who avoid anything that smacks of sadness in favour of the positive and – well, almost jolly. However, tango's emotional territory is not reserved for gloom. The musician and band-leader Enrique Rodriguez was criticised for his tendency to stick to the cheerful, as well as for an eclectic approach that saw his orchestra emerge as a budget, all-purpose band of jobbing professionals, able to turn out a foxtrot or a shimmy as well as a tango, often with the added sweetness of the singer Armando Moreno, his honeyed tones enriched, as one dance partner put it, with a Sinatra-like nicotine burr.

I am still learning about the singers. There is much to discover. Sometimes I recognise the velvet voice of tenor Raúl Berón sliding like a caress across time and distance to slip into the space between us; a poignant tremor, a soft touch on the skin. 'He's been dead forty years, I should think,' John says. 'What would he say if he could see us dancing to this now?' Recently I was delighted by what I heard as a choir of angels as I danced to the last song of a set. Enquiring later, I discovered there were only two voices, both male – perhaps there is something about the power of music that pushes us beyond the constraints of reality?

Then there are questions of weight and pace. Tango music as a whole contains three distinct strands, each with a different rhythm: tango itself, the waltz-time *vals* and, emerging from an earlier folk tradition, the *milonga*. Over time, the term 'milonga' came to mean the place where folk music could be heard and, gradually where one could dance. (Christine Dennsiton notes that Francisco Canaro in his autobiography claimed to have invented the term 'tango milonga' to describe a tango written for dancing.[3]) Eventually, the word became a shorthand for the event itself. The *milonga* dance, faster and more playful than a traditional tango, zips along to a pronounced two-beat rhythm. It presents its own challenges: to keep the feet tidy, not to bob up and down, and to stay with the music. As always, there is that tension between core strength and a relaxed posture, and the added trickiness of the *traspié*, literally a 'stumble step', a cross-rhythm which can be a delight if you manage it, or a repeated wrong-footing if not. It is above all else fun: the final notes are often lost in the laughter of those who have made it to the end without disaster. While the *milonga*'s giddy and hectic nature makes it particularly difficult for someone with Parkinson's, I was discovering that there were often occasions when it was the only thing that worked. When my feet dragged through a slow tango, my shoulders alternately twitching and stiffening, and I was beginning to think I would have to admit defeat and return to my seat, the impossible demands of the *milonga* would feel like an electrical charge, waking up nerve endings, switching on responses. The *vals* requires a different approach, asking for lightness from the dancer, for precision and fluency of step. While I struggled to achieve these qualities consistently, I loved to be asked, and discovered an immense pleasure in pushing through the lumpen heaviness of my condition.

At the other extreme, the music of Osvaldo Pugliese, bandleader, composer and pianist, asks for weight. I relish its richness and muscularity, its changes in tempo and pitch, and its intensity. His music was most popular in the industrial areas to the south of the Buenos Aires, where it echoed the sounds and rhythms of the machines in the factories. For the dancer, this is challenging territory. Although its dramatic qualities make Pugliese's music a favourite choice for show-tango, for me it recalls that last hour or so in the clubs and milongas in Buenos Aires, the sense of waiting for the Pugliese *tanda** eventually fulfilled as couples move onto the floor for this slower, more intimate dance. (While other orchestras may feature two

---

* In the milonga, songs are usually grouped in sets of three or four by the same orchestra, separated by a short piece of non-tango music — a *cortina* or 'curtain' — signalling that it's time to clear the floor and choose a different partner.

or even three times in an evening, Pugliese's challenging music tends to be played once only, late in the event, when all but the most dedicated (or addicted!) dancers have left and there is bit more space on the floor; as a result, it has a special quality.) At the beginning of my last visit, I promised myself I would manage a Pugliese set before I returned to England. On our final night at Club Gricel, as the first unmistakable notes filled the air, I grabbed the opportunity and – well, I managed. The music seemed to demand something more from the dancer – I wasn't sure exactly what, although I sensed it requires every ounce of energy and concentration, patience as the pauses linger, agility as the pace quickens. Back in Cambridge we often made time for Pugliese's music in the individual lessons – exhausting but exhilarating. As the phrases scratched and crackled, raw and urgent, veering from heights to depths and back, I felt they mirrored the sudden dipping and soaring of my spirits. And this is music you simply can't ignore. Even at my most sluggish and resistant, its challenge is irresistible: *You can't do this*, it says, *so go for it, do it anyway*.

The ending of a Pugliese piece follows the traditional pattern, that two-note finish that suggests both resolution and afterthought. 'Tum *tum*,' Alejandro in San Telmo murmured. 'Sol *doh*,' John said, after learning that they were the fifth and first notes of the scale, the dominant and tonic. 'Chan *chan*' is apparently the tango musicians' version. Some orchestras play the notes very softly; sometimes the last note seems not to be there at all. If that's the case, they say, listen more carefully; it's there somewhere. I like the ambiguity here: the song is over and not over. If there is a singer, the voice stops short of these two notes. The lingering instrumental finish suggests that at some level the dance is not really, not quite, over either.

Beginnings are significant, too. The convention on the dance floors of Buenos Aires is that the first bars of a piece are for listening, for familiarising yourself with what the music is asking, but also for a few moments' conversation with your partner. (Only tourists begin to dance as soon as the music starts.) This courtesy extends to the *cabeceo*, the unspoken invitation – a glance, a nod – so that new partners meet on equal terms at the edge of the floor. This is a risk: a prospective partner may have watched me dance, but he may not have realised that I have Parkinson's any more than I know how he will feel to dance with. The *cabeceo* is a leap in the dark, then, a statement of faith that in some way we will be able to make a nice dance together; that anything is possible.

Lesson notes
Our last lesson before the summer is crowded with memories: those first-time nerves, flowers on the table, the hiss of heavy rain through open windows, the day we talked so much we barely got started, side-tracked by poetry, anecdote and translation. And what's this got to do with tango? Or Parkinson's? Or teaching and learning? Everything.

This morning's lesson feels like a celebration, as well as an ending. We look for explanations for the way my troublesome right arm seems to be behaving itself. Perhaps I've had more sleep? Less stress? A growth in confidence? In fact, I believe it simply marks the progress we have made together. We begin with 'Tres Esquinas', a song from the 1940s. Three Corners – like Five Points – like in 'Gangs of New York', I say. The first few steps feel a bit stolid – in fact, so slow to start that John asks if the floor is sticky – but by the end of the first song I begin to feel the energy, the ability to move, filtering through to where my feet meet the ground. We dance a few tangos in close embrace. It feels comfortable, sweet, in tune; the occasional clunk, a few times when my foot catches in the floor or steps away too far, but mostly it feels good. 'A bit more pivot,' John says – and again: 'A bit more pivot.' '*Corazón* – the heart,' he says. As always, I am distracted by the words – *ojos* and *manos* (eyes and hands) and *recuerdo* (memory or souvenir). '*Sentimental*. What's that?' he asks. The same, I say. Although this may seem like lack of concentration, in fact it feels like the opposite: total focus on the music and its lyrics, ourselves, what we can achieve between us. The tangents – that Hotel Victoria story surfacing again – work rather to cement the common ground between us, a kind of extra layer to the music lapping around and over us as we work.

'Ten minutes in open embrace.' For the most part I am able to remain in my axis, upright, balanced, confident, stepping and pivoting. Three weeks earlier I couldn't have done this – in fact, I had been certain I could manage dancing in a close embrace only because of the secure support it offered, convinced that open embrace inevitably meant wobble and panic. Back to the close embrace: John suggests we focus now only on the music, setting aside other considerations. He begins to clarify: 'The music…' – but the explanation tails off – 'Well, you know…' Increasingly, meanings in these sessions are implicit: we have become so much in tune over the last six or seven months that common ground can be taken for granted. We dance. I listen, trying to catch the humour and delicacy of the song in my response. 'It's light,' we agree. Then a complete contrast: the uncompromising opening bars of Pugliese's 'Mariposa' – Butterfly, I translate. John nods, patiently: he knows, of course. Somehow we miss the first half of the song, chattering. We dance the second half then start the whole thing again. This is harder music for me; I don't know how else to explain it. It is heavy where the other piece was light, and then becomes deliciously light when you least expect it, changing tempo. I have to dig deep to find the energy to do it justice, but how satisfying it is when I feel I am its match.

We discuss plans for the next course of group lessons and whether it will contain enough challenge for me now, and I suggest the analogy of developing readers helped by independent readers: the learning cuts two ways, in that both benefit, though the analogy falls down at the point where tango, unlike reading, can never be a solo activity.

As for partners, I am gradually building a bank of leaders whom I can often rely on to dance with me, but my uncertainty and that charmed circle of better dancers mean it is slow progress. 'You need to be dancing with all and sundry,' John says. It's true. The catch is, I suppose, that as I become more accustomed to dancing with John, that confidence doesn't come as easily when I'm with others. There is also a long summer ahead, with the prospect of a double – or is it triple? – house move and a trip to France to visit friends, and for most of it I will be out of range of tango and, particularly, of John. How will I manage? How will this impact my health and well-being? I have certainly formed an attachment to John, one that's personal as well as practical – in the weeks before I left for Argentina, I felt a bit like a duckling imprinted on his tango shoes. So the celebrations are tinged with sadness and some trepidation, though I know that I'll have to stand on my own two tango feet eventually.

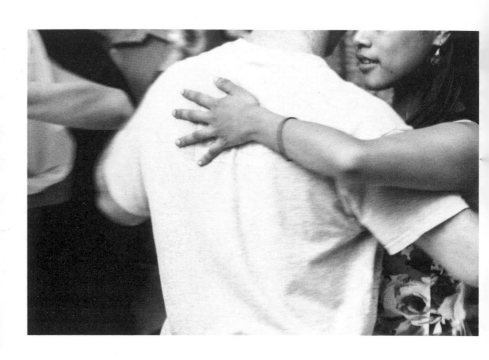

August:
Postcards II

Hallbankgate, Cumbria
Aches and pains. Packing. Other worlds. Rain.

'You will come to a time when everything hurts': I've always thought this line is from W. H. Auden's 'Atlantis' – except, when I check, it isn't; nor, indeed, is it anywhere else, apparently. But it's a line that has been lodged in my head for years. Did I invent it? In any case, it's not that everything hurts so much as a general, low-level ache and stiffness, joints and muscles that tense and jump without warning, a back that refuses to hold up, a background thumping head. Almost two weeks without tango; even the music has been shoved to the back of the queue by the imperatives of sorting, throwing, packing. When I finally manage to pick a route through the piles of dusty books and old photos to the CD player, the phrases sound thin. Where is the sustaining quality I need? If I could discipline myself to claim a mental space as well as a physical one, and practise, just walking (which, after all, is the basis of tango), twenty minutes' technique, or even a bit of yoga . . . But I'm too aware of the short time before my son and I have to leave the house which has been our home for the past twelve years. Given its situation, in a remote corner of north-east Cumbria, it has proved difficult to rent out, so the chance of a prospective tenant is too good to miss, despite the inconvenience that she wishes to rent the house unfurnished. My Cambridge house-hunting has so far drawn a blank. Somehow, I need to find somewhere not just for me to live, but to accommodate the accumulated possesssions of our small family.

Worlds rub up against each other. I've been reading Edmund de Waal's *The Hare With Amber Eyes* – in part an exploration of collecting – while we're absorbed in divesting, ridding. Cool wind blows in off the fell, under pale skies.

After two days of continuous rain, the air a dismal tippling, tatters of cloud hang low and the track outside the house has become a delta of brown, watery wastes separated by dwindling islands of grit and mud. This morning no rain as yet, but a stern sky suggests it won't be long. Inside, boxes and dust. Tango feels like ancient history. Four months ago I was writing postcards home from Argentina. Almost ten years earlier, I took my first tentative steps into the tango pool in the old school hall in Brampton, a couple of miles from here. On ancient varnish compacted by the footprints of hundreds of Cumbrian children, we were a collection of the odd and curious and accidental, all long legs and big bellies and anxious smiles. In the strong hands of Francis from Peebles (or was it Perth?) we practised our panther walk and tried out new moves until we thought we had it cracked.

Since then, I've gone back to the start several times over; a sense that the learning has only just begun. I'm reminded of a novel[1] in which the narrator, Lionel, describes his early tango experiences, in particular the challenge of intimacy, being in such close proximity to other people.

Just now, stranded briefly on this soggy shore, intimacy seems a faint memory: we might as well be at the other end of the known world.

Cambridge
Packing, Phase Two. Light on the Cam. Memories. Nomads.

A rash of birthdays is followed by packing sequence Phase Two, this time at the riverside flat in Cambridge, my temporary home in recent months. A later dawn than on the Cumbrian fellside I left yesterday, almost exactly twenty-three years since I arrived in Carlisle with my new husband on an unpromising Sunday afternoon in late summer. We were recently returned from Mexico, innocents in the worlds of Eighties Britain (one friend wrote about the problem of having too much cash – so they'd bought a second house – or was it a dishwasher?) and being married. Eventually we found somewhere to eat, the big place next to the

Cumberland News offices, which has changed hands several times since then. Could it have been called the Krakatoa? Yes, opened in '87, apparently, but it is now history. I expect it was raining.

I arrived back here in Cambridge yesterday afternoon, wearied by the weight of sorting and packing the accretion of *stuff* with which we seemed to have surrounded ourselves in Cumbria – a well-made wooden bed, roomfuls of fabrics fashioned into clothes and curtains, the brown rug from Chihuahua, bowls and bowls of stones, jars (yes, plural) of marbles never played with, endless drawers of schoolwork, mine and Jack's, and photos and letters . . . I have contrary urges to scoop the lot into a skip or to hang on to what seems most precious or necessary, so in the end I find an unsatisfactory middle way. At a car boot sale we sell a pair of iPods for £3.

Now, a perfect morning for last days: the palest blue sky, a washed-out circle of moon over the boathouses, a chorus of gulls offering a seaside illusion. If I look through the clustered lime leaves, Cambridge's heavenly summer scent long gone, I see light on the water. If I wait, there will be a cyclist on the far bank, and an out-of-season eight smoothing by. I am interrupted by echoes of other mornings: the day we walked up out of Caernarvon into the hills for a week's hiking in Snowdonia (we gave up after three days of constant rain). That was almost fifty years ago. A couple of years before that, I had sat on low steps in a suburban Midlands garden around dawn, with black coffee and an illicit cigarette, to make my goodbyes. This morning, I had thought to take my tea down on to the river bank. Instead I sit here and try to collect what seems important, charting my own journey into memory. I recall our last meal in our local, the Belted Will but always known simply as 'the Belted' back in Hallbankgate, three days ago. My son and I sat beside a party of shooters loud in their checked shirts, Jack brashly at home, me perched on the edge in my usual manner. I think of the day we moved in to the tiny house on Store Terrace, opposite the pub, Jack lodged somewhere out of the way for the day. His dad and I, newly separated, sat in front of the fire in the bar on that dour January night, chewing our way through a fish and chip supper, a reward for our two teenage movers, who ate silently next to us. We watched through the window for the lamps in the porch of number two to go dark, so that we would know when the previous owners had left and I could walk across the road to my new home.

'So, you've become a nomad?' David the car mechanic from the end of the track said, as he stepped forward for an unexpected and delicately formal farewell hug; in oily overalls, with his wall eye, the gentlest man.

Landroanec, Brittany
Sounds and silence. The piano. Histories. Swimming.

Murmuring pigeons; a muted clatter from the recently transformed cottage where Di is attempting to sort things into cupboards. The new rhythm of these days: a car passing nearby, a child's voice, the constant hiss of wind through pine and poplar. The Lac de Guerlédan shines silent through the trees. The space in front of the house – heaps of stone and broken tarmac, ditches, piles of breezeblocks – is also quiet, a hiatus of enforced calm after weeks of anxious packing.

I've been trying by telephone to arrange storage and transport for the final stage of the Cumbria-to-Cambridge move, so far with no success. Even if I could get hold of anyone, I am worrying about the piano. It's a heavy, double-stringed upright encased in a battered walnut veneer, and it's been in our family since before I was born. The story goes that when my dad was a boy growing up in a village near Wigan, he came upon a man pushing the piano, on a bogie, up the hill towards the tip. He raced home to fetch his father, who bought it (with the wheels, presumably) for half a crown. Did his family somehow find the money for lessons? They must have done: he played all his life, sometimes by ear, I think, but he could certainly read music and he played the organ in our various churches – bits of Bach and Handel and all those Methodist hymns, rattled out with an exuberance that eclipsed the wrong notes. Both my parents loved Gilbert and Sullivan, and Dad's signature piano piece was the overture to *The Mikado*. Some years after his death, I took my mum to see a production in Newcastle. As those first familiar notes rang out – *po-o-om* – *pa* – *pom-pom-pom-pom* – we glanced at each other with teary eyes and snivelled our way to the interval.

The piano is also the one I learned on. After I moved away, it lived for a while with family friends before it found its way home. Since then it's followed me round the country – and remained intact, apart from its pretty brass candlesticks, removed by my mum in a fit of 1950s modernisation. It's never quite in tune but it's become near enough a family member, which perhaps explains why it seemed necessary, although we had visitors, to spend an hour or two of our last Hallbankgate days downloading the words and sheet music for Kristina Olsen's 'My Father's Piano'.[2] Jack played, those big chords rolling around emptying rooms. Along with our old friend Nicky, we stumbled through a verse or two, to a bemused audience of Nicky's friends.

Here, now: one of those perfect French mornings, mist clearing over rolling fields, the air washed after another improbably deep sleep. In the distance, a dog barks. Soon it will be time for a pre-breakfast dip in the lake.

I finished *The Hare With Amber Eyes* – such a powerful book. I loved the pictures: photos, line drawings, maps. The book explores ways in which our possessions become a kind of family map, so that the Nazis' dismantling and destruction of the Ephrussis' collections reduces their precious belongings to just so much stuff. Without this geography – the map wiped clean, your sense of belonging gone – you become rootless, forced into a nomadic existence.[3]

My family history, pianos aside, is dull and domestic, about as far removed from great wealth or devastating Nazi brutalities as it could be, but I can identify with the sense of a tenuous connection to place, in my case stemming from a reluctance to be tied; what Michael J. Fox has called a 'keep-your-head-down-and-keep-moving mentality'. Here is Fox on what he calls one of the 'great ironies' of his life:

> … only when it became virtually impossible for me to keep my body from moving would I find the peace, security, and spiritual strength to stand in one place. I couldn't be still until I could – literally – no longer keep still.[4]

Lots of water yesterday: a magical early swim, warmish water under chill air, the mist sinking and settling over the lake as we entered, a lambency on the slopes on the opposite shore, and on the wall of a house. The surface of the water was streaked with bubbles, which multiplied as we swam, appearing magically in front of our moving arms, some as big as tennis balls. Then, in the afternoon, after a failed attempt to manage a bike with a crossbar and cycle into Mûr-de-Bretagne with Di, a trip to the far end of the lake in the boat, Nick at the helm, and hot chocolate (with cream) on the terrace at the Merlin before chugging home.

I'm looking well and feeling healthier here: the air and diet and exercise seem to suit me, although the bike incident was a reminder of the growing list of things I can't do, and I'm faintly horrified to recognise the soreness around my diaphragm as muscle strain from unwonted use – this in one who, a year ago, was swimming twice a week. (Time to set that right, once I'm back in Cambridge.) Here, I'm very aware of the stiffness and the aches and pains that trouble me less when I'm dancing regularly – I need to get back to tango as soon as I can. As with writing, there's the usual disquiet: will I have forgotten how?

> *Moving is the best medicine.*
>
> – Advert: Arthritis Foundation

I woke this morning to a sore back and pain down my left leg. As usual, it eases as I get up and move around. Meanwhile, the other kind of moving looms: Jack is rattling round in an empty Hallbankgate house, supervising Tuesday's furniture collection. I leave Landroanec later today for Poole and a couple of nights with Linda. She and I met on our first day at UCL in 1968 – we were roomed together in College Hall. I have never asked for her first impressions, but mine were distinctly dubious: she seemed much younger and more innocent, strait-laced and law-abiding, while I thought myself so grown-up, so modern, every inch a rebel. We have been close friends ever since. After Poole, a train back to Cambridge, where Mario and his team will arrive in the evening with the contents of Store Terrace. One more week of sofa-sleeping (back on my brother's couch!) before I finally shift into Albert Street, my new Cambridge home.

Will we swim this morning? The last few mornings have felt autumnal: chill air and a low sun. It's been a hard and slow process to warm up afterwards. But there is such magic in early light on a rippling surface, or disturbing a glassy calm, the stuff silky against the skin. Two days ago we dodged thundery showers and gales for a four-hour stroll around Cap d'Erquy, high cliff paths, gorse and heather, wild flowers and butterflies, small coves peeling back their white sand and turquoise sea as we rounded a corner.

No sun yet today.

Cambridge
Arrival. Transitions. Optimism.

Two days into Albert Street, the paint drying, stuff being housed bit by bit. This morning, Cumbrian weather.

A week and two days into back-in-Cambridge, the furniture into and out of storage thanks to one Bobby with a van, a week since my first tango lesson in John's new house in Histon Road. And almost a week since a weekend in Norfolk, missing a major tango event in an attempt to recover strength and health; and a day after tension exploded into a banging headache and dramatic vomiting –

an exact reprise of moving into my house in Cumbria, I recalled as I retched.

'Transitions' was the theme of Monday's yoga class, to the tune of Coldplay's 'The Scientist', Bombay Dub Orchestra's 'The Greater Silence', Bach's Prelude in C (on the piano) and Nina Simone's 'Feeling Good'. The teacher spoke about her eighty-year-old half-Italian mother moving sensually along Cambridge pavements with her feet firmly on the ground. We practised spreading our toes, feeling the strength of our roots. We thought about the transition from pose to pose, curl to stretch, fluency and grace. In tango, I thought, we work constantly with the transition from alone to together, stillness to movement, step to step. Against a background of the new term, the changing season, we laid out our own experiences of change; for myself, from hill country to flat, from the familiar to the new, from rain to sun (I hope). I left with a sense of well-being and optimism, a sensation that long-stifled creativity will have space to grow here.

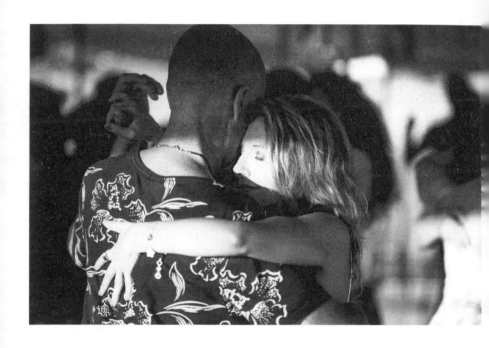

September:
Intimacy

The intimacy between two tango dancers can be intensified
when a community is dancing together, moving around the
room as a unified herd, pulsing in synchrony with the music.
Although the primary relationship in the dance rests with your
current partner, the connectedness that develops within a group
of dancers who respect others' space while ensuring flow around
the line of dance generates additional energy to be enjoyed by
all. Even watching the dance floor can be mesmerising.

— Ellie

The favoured facial expression for early dancers of Argentine
tango, and adopted by ballroom tango as the standard, was the
cara fea (ugly face), the stony mask devoid of feeling. Looking in
the mirror, sometimes I saw signs of the 'mask' associated with
Parkinson's, where the facial muscles lose mobility. Arriving
at a milonga, though, a glance at the faces of dancers as they
passed revealed closed eyes and blissful smiles, recalling Oliver
Sacks' description of the emotional awakening[1] that music can

effect, especially in those for whom feeling has become locked in or lost. It was as if tango cracked apart my Parkinson's face, uncovering and releasing the joy I found in my core.

Just about all the tango lyrics I can think of contain the word *corazón* – the heart. Many are built around the central heart motif: the bruised heart, the beating heart, the heart that is torn between two lovers, or between two countries, or that belongs only to the mother, or to the one who will never return the love, or to 'you'. In Federico Silva's lyrics to 'Amor de Verano' ('Summer Love'), for example, the singer remembers a time when 'every night was a dawn, every dawn a caress, every kiss a song', when he and his lover were so close that, although they were two, they became one – '*un corazón*'. The music is sometimes heavy with longing, though often with a lightness of touch that delights. This is no accident: in Buenos Aires, tango is danced with intensity, full-bodied and full-blooded. Sexy? Not really – or rather, yes, sometimes, but not in any obvious way. Although my body is almost as close to my partner's as it is possible to get, the physical nearness is merely the starting point. So, passionate, then? Well, kind of: this is what they always say about tango, but the word suggests to me those individuals who dance for display, often hurriedly, leaving the partner behind in their urgency to discover or reflect this elusive quality. Real passion is embedded deep within the connection between dancers, but there is little pleasure in dancing with a leader who is really dancing only with, and for, himself.

The heart is a wonderful metaphor. The other day I came across a T-shirt saying 'I love REALISM', where 'love' is represented by a lump of red muscle rather than the love heart in the 'I love NY' logo. The neat irony makes me smile, but tango similarly works on two levels: the heart symbolises love, affection, emotion, but in tango you are also close enough physically to feel your partner's heartbeat, to be aware of two hearts beating as one, as the poets say. Between-songs chat – *chamuyo* – on Buenos Aires dance floors, delicately framed so that considerations of wealth or status or employment are tactfully excluded, leans toward the emotional: 'Here we dance with the heart' or 'I love this song'. Often the conversation will be laced with *piropos* (compliments) – an 'unforgettable' dance is a good example – according to Francesca all part of 'the theatre of the milonga'. Accuracy matters less than intention, a willingness to open yourself to the music, your partner, the dance.

So what does this have to do with Parkinson's? As far as I know, although the brain has stopped functioning properly, the heart is unaffected by the condition. And fortunately for people like me, to dance tango is not about remembering figures, nor concentrating on a pre-agreed sequence of moves. It works best when I manage to stop thinking altogether and… just dance.

Tango begins with an invitation to get up really close, so it is fitting that the approach is made sensitively, discreetly, from a respectful distance. According to convention, the man invites, the woman responds, although who is to say who makes the first move in the unspoken *cabeceo*? Opinion is divided on this. Some believe that the system reflects a *macho* culture where women sit separately and passively until summoned by a man. Others feel that the opportunity to respond, or not, before a leader approaches directly, or to choose a leader for yourself, is empowering. Certainly an unspoken agreement made with a glance across the floor can be preferable to the sudden arrival in front of you of a prospective partner, particularly if you would prefer not to dance at this point. Having some experience of dancing in Buenos Aires, where the *cabeceo* is in many cases the norm, a direct approach feels like an intrusion into my personal space.

As soon as I walk onto the floor, though, I accept that my personal space will be shared both with the other couples and, most obviously, with my partner. We stand directly in front of each other, exchanging a look, perhaps a smile or a greeting. The first twenty or thirty seconds of the song may be given over to chatting, allowing the music to suggest how we might move. Then the leader offers his left hand, open, palm facing. In return I offer my right hand and then my body. While it is possible to dance tango at a distance, in an 'open' or partially open embrace, for me tango is essentially a dance of close embrace: what is sometimes described as a natural, loving hug. There is an equality in this embrace: both leader and follower offer and accept only as far as they wish or are able. We adjust. His right arm moves round my back, until I feel the palm of his hand, or perhaps the lower edge of the palm, against my spine. My left arm rests lightly on his shoulder or upper back so that there is a firm but light contact between our upper arms. As we hear the opening bars of the song, we breathe together. I listen for his intention. In an ideal world, rather than rushing to start, we wait for that connection before we begin.

On a purely physical level, this close encounter can be a challenge. Non-tango friends are often squeamish about being up so close to all those *men*. And there can be issues, I suppose, around smell, for instance. Some people do smell, and not just of soap or aftershave (though there are some who smell faintly, tantalisingly delicious). Some sweat a lot, so there is a kind of subculture of the towel-and-quick-change-of-T-shirt variety. Sometimes a *tanda* in a warm hall will result in a damp frock or in hair stuck to your face. In practice, such things matter very little because so many other aspects of closeness are more important. There are certainly no secrets, though: for our 'twelve minutes of love'[2] we may be separated only by a couple of layers of thin fabric. My partner may well find himself with an armful of twitch and jitter, or an upper body as hard and unresponsive as a girder. Often these initial tics will fade, but it only takes an impatient tug at my jiggling hand to exacerbate the problem. And just try telling me to 'relax'! Yet in the same way that any relationship is a statement of faith, stepping into the tango embrace requires an acceptance of risk. If I hold back, nothing works. Settling for half won't do.

Here I am, I am saying, with my imperfections, anxieties, preoccupations. This is the shape I am, the person I am and also the person I aspire to be. Be patient. Don't rush to judge, or to defend yourself. I won't criticise you or compare you to other partners. For these minutes let's be open to each other and to the music and see what we can make of it.

The benefits of opening oneself in this way are huge, particularly for an individual with Parkinson's, where the psychological and emotional repercussions of the disease often prove more difficult than the physical symptoms. Although I hadn't yet reached the stage where I felt 'locked in' by the condition, a sense of isolation had become a recurrent hazard. I was the same person as I used to be, yet different. Preoccupation with energy levels or balance, frustration with fumbling fingers or a tripping foot, often threatened an already precarious sense of worth. Because the symptoms felt too minor, too tedious to discuss, I would try to hide them and in doing so would feel the gap between myself and others only widen. Close contact with another human being, contact which feels safe, respectful and equal, is a powerful counter to alienation and despair. As a single person with the condition, I experienced being held as a precious gift, offering the validation I often struggled to find for myself.

For those of us lucky enough to dance in its supportive and democratic community, tango can provide a model for relating to others in the world beyond the milonga: an openness and acceptance, and an opportunity for mutual support. Rather like the bypass system that tango seems to create in the damaged brain, involvement in the dance enables us to bypass class, education and the day-to-day so that we are able to connect with one another at a deeper level and on an equal basis. The sense that a partner and I could move together in response to the music in a way that transcended self-consciousness or common sense was an extraordinary experience, and a moving one.

Of course, intimacy is a risky business and the emotional risks are played out in tango on a physical level. The use of 'disassociation', where my hips turn away from my partner while my chest stays with him, suggests ambivalence: I want to be close but I also want to move away. In the *sacada*, the leader literally takes away the follower's space. In the *gancho*, one partner fleetingly inserts a leg between the legs of the other to execute a 'hook'. And for the *volcada*, the leader briefly overturns or capsizes the axis of the follower, stealing her balance before restoring it. The conventional physical boundaries that we take for granted in our cold, British way – keep your distance, respect others' personal space – are flouted at every turn. With more practice at trusting my partner and the process, I became more confident that what was taken would be repaid and the equilibrium recovered. As a dancer with Parkinson's, figures like these made light of my difficulties in a creative way, unseating me where I was most insecure but offering me reassurance that, as for any other dancer, order would be quickly restored.

As well as addressing motor ability, then, tango can provide the experience of intimacy, particularly precious where intimacy in the 'real' world has become problematic – hence the belief that therapies which address both motor and affective issues are more useful for people with Parkinson's than those which focus entirely on the physical aspects of the condition. Rather than merely a therapeutic dose of intimacy, though, I had been blessed with the real thing, which extended beyond the dance floor. While John and Ellie always maintained the highest professional standards in their teaching, much of the healing that I was experiencing stemmed from their readiness for risk, and the strength of their friendship.

A friend with a condition such as Parkinson's, where psychological and emotional well-being are fragile to say the least, can be a bit of a liability, as Ellie and John discovered to their cost. As the illness became more difficult to manage, they both found themselves on the receiving end of sound and fury from me. I suppose I could claim a similar courage: opening myself to the extent that I had done, I made myself vulnerable. In one lesson, looking for a way to reduce tension and rigidity in my upper body, we practised keeping the weight down around the hips, our hands lower and looser. 'This will help you to relax your shoulders, to be more responsible for your own axis, less dependent on me,' John said. Was I becoming overdependent emotionally, too? A reading at a local festival celebrating the work of Virginia Woolf reminded me that we must 'face the fact, for it is a fact, that there is no arm to cling to, but that we go alone'.[3]

Lesson notes

Several weeks since our last lesson and Kate is a little rusty. The back steps are hesitant and the balance in open embrace is unreliable, but once she starts to relax and warm to the class, things improve. Then she tells me that she's been having trouble getting downstairs and can't get on her bike, which is hard to believe after seeing her dance. But in the dance she feels the partner's embrace, she knows she won't fall, and the music provides a sort of reference for where and when she should be. Under these conditions there is a transformation in her confidence which allows her to move naturally and elegantly. This MUST be good for her because, as long as she doesn't forget how it feels to move naturally, I think she won't stop being able to do so.

— John

The sleep problem, I know, is widespread. It is a particularly common aspect of Parkinson's and is becoming more the norm than the exception for me. I never know how best to deal with it, particularly when it matters: in sixteen hours' time I want to be able to dance beautifully until midnight. This feels especially important since I haven't made it to a milonga for a while and we've had some encouraging lessons. How will I be able to remain upright if I haven't slept? But I've spent enough nights turning over determinedly and checking the clock every hour to know that this doesn't work either. So here I am, just before five o'clock in the morning, with no sign of dawn, drinking tea and thinking about yesterday's lesson.

I didn't tell John how low my spirits had plummeted after our good lesson the previous week. Now, I can put it down to the toll that the multiple house moves took on my well-being, physical and emotional; to the continued upheavals, the rain, and not being able to settle to write... I felt as if I'd pushed my father's piano — was still pushing it — up a long, slow incline. So it was easy to convince myself, when I didn't hear from John for a few days, that he'd had enough. Ten minutes into the lesson, though, I am reminded that he is still here, and that I can dance. He offers some praise, albeit tongue-in-cheek — 'All right, that's an "A" now' — but what really works is that the lesson enables me to do well at what we have been practising for months. Incredibly, in these troubled times, I can sense improvement, even on last week. Today we pay attention to detail: the exact length and placing of the side step in the *giro*, the timing and strength of the *boleo*, the mechanics of the *volcada*. It's great: absorbing, instructive and supportive. It works. I get it. I know now what I have achieved — and what I can't do yet, what I need to practise.

For me, though, this is only a small part of the benefit. Expert and patient always, John is also John, and this is what he brings to our lessons: the whole, real person. We talk, for example, about some of his uncertainties about teaching.

He trusts me enough to share these with me. After almost half a lifetime teaching English to eleven- to eighteen-year-olds, this is an area where I am strong, so the process really does feel mutual and equal. I need this. I believe it is exactly this affirmation of worth and friendship that keeps me hopeful, forgetting the bloody *thing* and remembering that I, too, am a whole person and probably an OK one after all – and, sometimes, for moments, I can dance quite beautifully. I recognise John's anxieties as the marks of a caring professional, ready to question or to rethink in order to work more effectively. This wakes me up to the fact that my condition is not the only thing we're grappling with here. All of us struggle with whatever we're up against, to find a way to make the best we can out of whatever we have or don't have, and tango is (again, and always) both an opportunity to do this and a model for the other, disparate, bits of our lives.

So there we are. Yesterday I thought about mirrors – the two large ones in his teaching room – but also mirroring, the way many aspects of our lives have seemed to share a similar turmoil recently. In my new house, the boiler seems to have developed a trick, like his boiler, of starting up randomly through the night. I also hear an occasional dripping sound – or is it a chirping? An insomniac grasshopper in the woodwork? And then there is the piano, silent now but here, and on level ground.

Six a.m. Approaching daylight.

★

The lesson with you, Kate, was lovely as usual. It brought me into the moment and made me focus on every minute. I can enjoy dancing with you while at the same time thinking of how you could make it even better. I can feel the limits of where we have got to and can nudge at them a little until they shift to a new waterline. I think we need to keep pushing gently and see what happens… We have to make the best of what we have, but first we have to believe that what we have already is wonderful. That will give us much encouragement.

— John

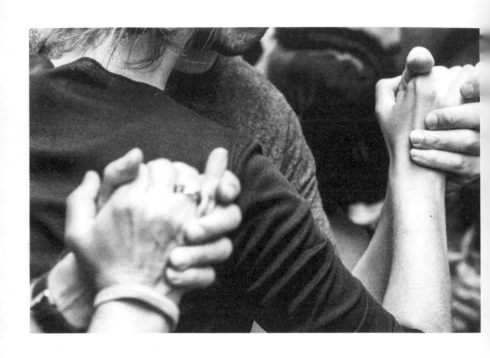

October:
Medicine

There's a postcard pasted to the side of my bookshelf – a print of William Blake's engraving of a human figure in a stormy sea. The man – I think it's a man – is looking upwards through the waves and has an arm raised vertically, stretched up to the dark sky, fingers splayed. It's called *Help! Help!* It lives in the Fitzwilliam Museum in Cambridge and I've seen the original. On a visit to the museum with my mum some years ago, I left her looking at nineteenth-century furniture while I wandered ahead and then up a steep and narrow spiral staircase to the balcony gallery of small prints and paintings, in search of works by Blake. What I found is lost in the memory of the panic I felt when I realised I couldn't attempt the staircase down again without help – not strictly a Parkinson's moment, although its pervasive insecurities with balance may well have added to my tendency to vertigo when facing even the smallest of heights. Long minutes passed, both upper gallery and room below empty of other visitors. Eventually a man appeared in the doorway and I was able to call out and persuade him to climb the stairs so that I could follow him down. 'I thought you'd been rather a long time,' Mum said.

Sometimes what you need to ask for is as obvious as this, although the asking in itself is a challenge. It can be preferable to cower quietly out of the way and hope for a return of courage or some magical rescue. But there are benefits in approaching a stranger. As the last traces of the summer's warmth evaporated, I started to find myself embarrassed by my need – or was it neediness? I didn't know who or what to ask, or how or when. How late was too late? How much was greedy? How long before those closest to me felt the tug and chafe of me as a weight around their generous necks? I felt I should be able to manage. Now in my sixties, I was a mother, an ex-professional, clever, moderately healthy and solvent, with friends and family close by. What was it King Lear said? 'O, reason not the need!'[1] But he was old and desperate, and quite without the wisdom that age is supposed to give.

Autumn brought a consolidation of symptoms that had been intermittently troublesome for months, like a spell of bad weather setting in for the winter. In fact, the weather coincided with the arrival of dark days and long nights, the brief fling of a balmy Indian summer summarily translated into fringe hurricane weather, all sudden squalls and a troubled sky. In the lovely house, unpacking done, the oversized oven loomed: 'Cook me!' My digestive system took up a permanent state of protest. My ankles were nettled with fleabites from someone else's cat. I toppled off the bike into gutters, crashed sideways into doorways, woke in the too-early dark. Checkout operators sighed as I struggled to pack shopping. There was the promise of a cold sore on my upper lip, and what I thought might be RSI in my left arm. Nearly adrift, isolated, I clung on to flotsam. Was this tango deprivation, or evidence that the disease was moving towards a next stage? The tango medicine still worked, no question, but the effort it took to get to the place where energy levels were restored and movement eased was increasing, and increasingly too much to contemplate.

Discouraged, I looked for better medication of the pharmaceutical kind. The search took me from GP to consultant, the first neurologist I'd spoken to for five years. Why did I expect a man, and one my age? The doctor was tiny, impossibly young, and very pregnant. She ran through a list of questions, recording my answers carefully. She displayed polite interest in my tango tales. Rather than a stronger dose of my current medication, she prescribed a supplementary dopamine agonist to help the L-dopa to work better. At home later, I poked about on the internet looking for information on the new pills. The first side effect listed for dopamine agonists was euphoria. Unlikely? In fact the new medicine and I didn't hit it off. It had the effect of a blunt instrument to the head, rendering me stupid and even more sluggish. I was swamped by fatigue. Only a month or two to Christmas and I couldn't even manage a glass of wine without sinking into a near-coma. The product had a name so close to Rohypnol and its associations with 'date rape' that I found myself looking nervously over my shoulder. After four doses, I pushed the box to the back of the cupboard.

Was I losing faith in the healing power of tango? How could I recover the strong charge of those early days, when I felt I could almost manage without the drugs? On a previous visit to Argentina, I met a woman with Parkinson's for whom dancing tango spelled freedom, enabling her to set aside the wheelchairs, walkers and sticks she had needed to cope with her condition. She had evolved a hypothesis to explain the process: that the rhythmic frequency of tango music was decoded in the inner ear into nerve impulses that travelled through the body of the healthy dancer to the palm of his hand, where it would meet the hand of his partner. There this energy would be transmitted into her hand via her fingertips. Her theory continued with a discussion of electrical impulses, neurotransmitters and endorphins activated by the acoustic stimulus of the music, which would restore a healthier pattern of movement in the recipient. I wasn't sure whether it was the difficulty of translation or the difficulty of the science that confounded me. I wanted to understand this apparently magical process, wanted to believe in the possibility of such a radical transformation. Although it might sound more the stuff of New Age fantasy and wishful thinking than an objective reality, it did at least speak to the whole person. The world of medical professionals seemed to operate piecemeal, my symptoms becoming separate entities. I took my tremor and fatigue to the neurologist, my depression and insomnia to the GP, my digestive issues to the nurse, while the rest of me – the familiar muddle of bone and juice and dissatisfaction – remained untreated.

In the best traditions of holistic medicine, tango treated all of me simultaneously, and the discipline of the dance provided a structure within which I could work safely. Motor difficulties and muscular tension were addressed by the music, by the demands of the rhythm and by the lead of my partner. Struggles with balance were eased as I worked at core strength and maintaining my own axis in the support of the embrace. As well as physical benefits, the dance tackled the emotional and psychological aspects of the disease. The erosion of confidence was reversed, potentially, by the fact that I was able to achieve more than I could outside of tango. And the ever-present sense of isolation could be countered by the intimacy experienced in the dance. The intensity of the connection with my partner was strengthened by the connection between other couples who shared the dance floor. I was part of a series of concentric circles of support, held in the centre by my partner, by other couples on the floor with us, and by the wider tango community in this town, this country, worldwide. I also had my place in those circles, holding others in return.

Ellie once asked the question: how can the tango effect be bottled? Of course, tango is never going to be widely available on prescription, although a recent study recommends that dance become part of a 'comprehensive management plan' for people with Parkinson's, as it has 'the potential to target cognitive and emotional aspects of the disease in addition to the physical impairments'.[2] Certainly the benefits of tango, for all – healthy or otherwise – can be accessed regularly in most places relatively cheaply. In addition to what I gained from and contributed to the group, it seemed that continuing the regular one-to-one lessons operated like a booster dose, both workout and recuperation, a kind of physical and emotional realignment as well as an opportunity to practise my skills. On occasions when my confidence in the group situation foundered, this was my sustenance. It may be that, as I get older or the disease takes a stronger hold, individual sessions like these become the norm, but there are indications that neither age nor illness is a handicap in dancing In the short film *The Embrace of Aging*,[3] dance instructor Helaine Treitman describes her oldest pupil as her 'secret weapon', the favourite of every female dancer. And the many available YouTube videos of Osvaldo 'Honey Feet' Cartery and his wife and partner Coca show us the skill and mastery that the old *milongueros* spent a lifetime achieving.

Tango is often casually described as addictive. Did this account for what seemed like my growing tolerance to the drug? Did I need to increase the dose to achieve the same effect? How was this practicable when energy was the first casualty? How was it possible to sustain the impact of tango over time? And if addiction was a real possibility, could I overdose? For me, tango had come to represent the drive to take on challenges, to push past obstacles. It may be that this is not always the healthiest option. While the difficulties of the dance help the ageing or ailing brain to branch out, encouraging new growth, there may also be a need for acceptance – that, after all, not everything is always possible.

Lesson notes

On the way to the lesson, a fall – not from grace, but from the bike again. A bag of books for the Amnesty shop threatened to spill out of the basket as I wobbled along Bermuda Terrace, anxious to arrive on time. I put out a hand to catch Liddell Hart's huge tome, crashed into the cemetery railings and toppled sideways. Only bruises this time, although it made for an uncertain start to our hour. We worked on responses to subtler leads, on disassociation, then moved to *milonga*: how to keep the upper body still but relaxed, especially, in my case, the shoulders.

A couple of days later there is a workshop in Cambridge with Eric Jeurissen from Tango El Corte, in Nijmegen, though he is now just off a plane from New York. His class is called 'Surprise Me'. We dance to early recordings of Juan D'Arienzo's orchestra – a 1930s reaction against then current trends towards more elaborate, formal, salon tango, Eric explains, the emphasis of the music being fun. Eric is affable and encouraging. He notes at the start that, as a group, our dancing is mechanical and rather tired, but promises that by the end of the class we will have improved. He returns several times to his signature notion of 'finding the floor'. 'The floor is your friend,' he says. I watch with envy as a very self-possessed dancer crosses the room in flesh-coloured ballet pumps just before the class begins, each step landing firmly, as if it has found its home, in contrast to my jittery stance, where all my weight is somehow carried in my upper body.

We begin with a model for back *ochos* – two steps back then a back cross, moving to a tighter cross, then a back cross in the other direction. We are looking for energy in the dance: 100 per cent presence. The notion of surprise, that sudden reversal into the opposite back cross, is crucial in tango, Eric says. I think this is one of the factors that makes tango so difficult, but also so productive, for someone with Parkinson's. Responding to the unexpected impacts directly on that 'stuck' state that can occur: there is nothing for it but to go. A change of partners brings me to dance with John. Eric's intervention: 'Yes, be with him, but not like that; put your shoulders down.' He doesn't quite say the infuriating 'Just relax.'

The second figure is the front *ocho* – in fact, two front *ochos*, the third becoming a turn. We work on this individually, my initial panic (I can't do this without some support!) alleviated slightly by John's supportive presence. But of course I can manage, after a fashion, and a tip from the front creates a small epiphany: if you keep your chest turned to your notional partner as you begin the *ochos* and then turn into that space instead of turning away, it will be easier. It is. Eric tells us to practise at home. 'You must train yourselves to do this,' he says. I resolve to do so. He interrupts later when I am dancing with Mariusz, my main partner for the class. 'Find the floor, Kate,' he says, and (as he steps in momentarily), 'the lower you are, the easier it is for me to find you. Also breathe, breathe out now, from the belly.'

No new learning, then, but the boost of a fresh angle, a sense of progress made. For me, the importance of being firmly planted in the floor (remember all those weeks of the tree pose in yoga?) is a good counter to the intention to be 'up' in the dance, muscles engaged, rather than sagging. I need to work out how to get the balance right without carrying it all in my shoulders. If my centre of gravity is up there, is it any wonder I keep falling?

In a serendipitous way yesterday's yoga was focused on relaxing the shoulders. It was preceded by another fall, this time in the shower; nothing serious, though alarming. I think back to pre-diagnosis days and all those tumbles when out running, and also of the 'postural instability' (even the terminology is ugly) that is a feature of the P-thing. Even so, I don't just have to settle for this precariousness. I can work at 'finding the floor', and stop charging around in too much of a hurry. As well as tango, there are other ways I can 'break a sweat' (the only kind of exercise that counts, we are advised). This morning I go for a short run, the first in months, remembering to lift my feet like a circus pony to prevent my lazy right leg from tripping me on tree roots. On the way back, I make a doctor's appointment – time for another review of the medication; the non-tango medication, that is.

I find myself thinking about my dad again. He has blustered his way into my mind a number of times recently; something to do with moving that piano the length of the country, perhaps, or the fact that his photograph is on the wall here now. Christened Frederick but always Fred, he was much loved. He commanded huge respect from almost everyone he met for his boundless energy, his relentless enthusiasm, his drive to complete any project he started. Charismatic, compelling, he was also overwhelming. At times I found him insufferable, impossible to live with. A fiend for serious music, he would stand in the centre of the living room conducting as a Mahler symphony or Wagner's *Götterdämmerung* pounded out from the speakers. 'Listen,' he would say. 'Listen… Listen to this bit. Just listen.' I still find Wagner hard to stomach, but I know I've inherited more than just his love of music: my own passions can be very demanding. One of the last photos of we have of Fred was taken on his birthday, on the newly installed church roof, the Derbyshire countryside spread out beneath him. An engineer all his working life, the renewal of the roof was his final major project. He has company in the photograph, and of course he couldn't have completed the job on his own, but he got up there by himself. I'm reminded of the ladders in Joan Miró's paintings, opportunities for escape but also aspiration, 'as if one could climb up to the stars' as one reviewer of the Tate exhibition put it.[4] I'm aware that my own ladder to the stars has been rather wobbly of late, needing the steadying hands of those closest to me more frequently, but I haven't forgotten that before too long I have to learn to stand on my own two feet.

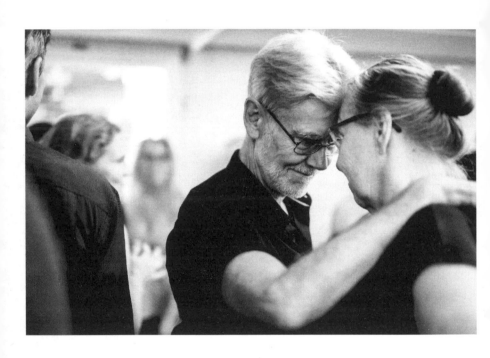

November: Communities

Over the course of the last year or so, I have puzzled how best to teach someone with Parkinson's. I have read about Parkinson's; I have tried to empathise with how Kate is feeling and what she has to do to make her body comply with her brain. I know that there have been classes organised by other dance disciplines especially for people with Parkinson's disease and benefits have no doubt been enjoyed, but one of our principles at Cambridge Tango is to create a welcoming and inclusive community.

— John

When I began this book, it was about me, the remarkable impact of Argentine tango on 'my' condition. It wasn't entirely selfish – I could envisage others benefiting from what I had learned – but the story I was telling was essentially my own. I don't think I ever lost sight of the huge contribution made by John and Ellie, or of the fact that for them, too, this was a process of discovery. But I certainly regarded myself as the main character.

Towards the end of the year news reached me that my favourite contemporary dance company, the Mark Morris Dance Group (based in Brooklyn but regularly touring worldwide), was running workshops for people with Parkinson's and their families, friends and care partners. I'd been a fan of the company since my first encounter with their work some years earlier, via a borrowed video of *Falling Down Stairs*, a collaboration with cellist Yo-Yo Ma, and I'd seen them several times in performance since. I discovered that since their Parkinson's outreach began in 2001, they now held classes in six venues in the New York area and through affiliated groups in over one hundred communities in sixteen countries around the world. Their aim: to ensure that 'each class is an aesthetic experience, integrating mind, body and emotion', allowing people with Parkinson's to experience the 'joys and benefits' of dance while addressing the specific symptoms of the condition – in particular, balance, cognition, motor skills, depression and physical confidence. The Mark Morris group believes its Dance for PD programme has been an 'important catalyst' in creating active, engaged Parkinson's communities where there were none, due in part to an 'inclusive philosophy that welcomes all, regardless of ability or level of mobility'.[1]

I liked the emphasis on community and inclusion, although this was a different inclusion from the one I was enjoying as an active member of tango communities in Cambridge and further afield. But I wasn't attracted either by specialist classses or by notions of 'tango therapy', where the dance was simplified into a series of exercises or treatments. Acceptance on an equal footing in a world where I was not defined by the condition had become an important factor for me in countering the emotional toll of Parkinson's, and I was keen to share the benefits with others. John, Ellie and I arranged a tango demonstration and taster session for a local Parkinson's group. Rather than a separate course for people with Parkinson's, we wanted to offer in-class support in our regular beginners' lessons and, eventually, supported attendance at milongas. This never got off the ground, however – even those who had seemed keenest during our demonstration didn't come forward to take part. Maybe we hadn't thought it through sufficiently at this stage. Or perhaps specialist courses are simply less daunting, for both provider and recipient. Still, I didn't want tango to be adapted or made easy for me. I wanted to meet the challenge of this most difficult of dances. While I was sure there were worthwhile and useful therapeutic programmes that included Argentine tango, I was holding out for tango in the real world, rather than tango therapy, for as long as I could.

An autumn visit to Barcelona to celebrate a birthday taught me some new lessons, not just about community but about the nature of tango iself. Rather like the Buenos Aires trip, this holiday was an opportunity – four nights' dancing and a chance to reconnect with old friends – but also a challenge. Would my stamina survive the journey, sleep deprivation and the inevitable high-octane eating and drinking? Would I be able to pick my way through the tangle of tripwire that Parkinson's might strew across the dance floor? Like any other *tanguera*, I hoped for that perfect tango, a dance with a stranger in which I might find the ultimate connection. And somewhere in the back of my mind was the possibility, the outside chance, that I might just meet someone looking for more than a dance partner, and to whom a sixty-something with a boxful of odd moves and a head of blonde curls might appeal.

'Be careful what you wish for': isn't that what they say? There was no tango romance, of course, but there were several living reminders of why I was glad to be single. And the perfect tango? No, although there were near-perfect moments: the ability to lose myself in the strong arms of old friends, and one or two moderately delicious encounters with local dancers at the Halloween special at La Yumba. (Was that really a *sentada*, or was the sense that I was sitting on his knee for a bar or two a way of overlooking a cheekier intention?) I survived a scramble round the floor with a giant of a chap in what I presumed was fancy dress – seamed stockings, stilettos, a set of foam rubber false breasts that bobbed around at (for me) eye level, and monster make-up, complete with an inventive repertoire of roars and growls. Or perhaps that was his usual weekend persona? At any rate, our group was welcomed in all the dance venues with generosity and patience, even though, as an influx of twenty dancers, we filled up every available chair and made for a very crowded milonga.

One advantage of Argentine tango is its global nature. In many cities across the world I could walk into a milonga as a single woman and be comfortable and safe. The international tango community operates a clear system of unspoken codes of behaviour: respect your partner, taking care of his or her safety; be entirely present and focused on the dance; and respect the other couples moving in the shared space with you. For this reason you keep to the line of dance, following the circular anticlockwise progression around the room, moving in a disciplined manner. Anything else, according to *milonguero* Santiago ('Santi') León, is 'tango fantasy'. Like any community, members look after each other. Rules about avoiding high kicks in a crowded space, for example, are there to protect its members. (Not everyone agrees.) Of course, there are leaders who dance to demonstrate their own prowess, sending their followers spinning in the centre of the floor, and teachers who show off their own perfect pivots at the expense of intervening to help their struggling students. I am surprised at every turn, though, by the active sense of responsibility for others that characterises an effective community.

Dancing with someone with Parkinson's has risks, from the minor embarrassments of fudged steps or sluggish feet to more obvious disasters. My first dance of our final milonga in Barcelona lasted all of thirty seconds, during which nothing worked: fuzzy head, balance shot, legs with no order or coherence; I could barely stay upright. I stumbled through an apology in Spanish, muttering something along the lines of 'maybe later' and subjecting myself and, worse, my partner, to the indignity of abandoning the attempt and leaving the floor. So I'm ready to forgive those leaders who won't risk it. But there are many who, week after week at home, or regularly on trips like this last one, are up for it. To those ready to embrace uncertainty or who know what to expect and come back for more, I am always grateful.

More than this, though, I was beginning to understand more of what tango is about, as well as what it isn't. First, it isn't an 'activity' that can be dismantled and repackaged in an easier 'therapeutic' version. For someone with a movement disorder such therapy might be suitable exercise, but it isn't tango. Also, like martial arts, tango is less about technique than about attitude. What is central is the connection with your partner, with the music, and with others who share the floor. Suddenly it made sense: partners such as Martin, Dave, John, Robert, Alan, Santiago, Donald and Derek are not heroes. They are the ones who get it. It is this amazing connection that's the point – not a *boleo*, not a well-executed *barrida*.

My first dance in Barcelona was with my Cumbrian tango teacher Lili's partner, Santi. I had arrived in the city in time to meet everyone for a late lunch in the Argentinian restaurant Nueve Reinas. We ate, drank, spent an hour or two wandering around the Fundació Antoni Tàpies; then a quick unpack, wash, change – and straight to 'Antonia's Milonga' for ten o'clock. We arrived at the tail end of a class. I have a hazy memory of a largish square room with a stage at one end, chairs with white covers, delicious music, and sitting long enough to decide that I might just make it to the bar but that I was too exhausted to think about dancing – when I found Santi standing in front of me. I don't know why I brushed aside Lili's whispered protective protest and hauled myself to my feet. Manners? Determination? I think there was a song and a half left in the *tanda*, and I managed it – no triumphs, no disasters. I still think of those six minutes or so with gratitude. 'Don't worry too much,' he said at the first stumble. He's a graceful, polished dancer who was then building a reputation and a career, very selective in his choice of partner, and this was a big risk for him: we'd barely met (though of course he knew my story from Lili) and he'd never seen me dance. For taking that risk, for his generosity and trust, I loved him instantly.

Predictably, our evenings in Barcelona ended with us sitting round the big table in the apartment picking over the milongas, discussing the dancing, the venue, new friends. We were a very mixed group and our conversations weren't only about tango. Over the six days I listened to detailed accounts of Roman battle re-enactments, the problems of a conifer hedge, the decision to abandon a career in entomology ('A particular kind of beetle,' he said apologetically) and a Cornish wedding. Santi tried to master 'How much wood could a woodchuck chuck…'; it didn't get easier after a glass or two. I remembered that one of the loveliest dancers in our group was a *Daily Mail* reader. But how incredibly fortunate we were: all this *stuff* was peripheral. What mattered was that tango enabled us to connect on a deeper level. Soul to soul, heart to heart might sound like a cliché, but try it and see.

So, our last night in Barcelona: 'Norma's Milonga', sometime after midnight. After giving up on the first dance, I spent an hour drinking water, watching, chatting. Martin appeared: tall, with that familiar mix of strong and gentle. We managed a lovely set, almost coming to grief on the last step but not quite. A few more dances, and then I saw Santi nod in my direction. I can't recall the music; I wonder if he remembers. But for me the whole *tanda* teetered on the edge of wonderful. 'Very nice,' he said – surprised, perhaps – after our first song together. I was still glowing as we left. In the doorway, I was approached by the man I had abandoned on the dance floor at the start of the evening. 'We didn't get our dance after all,' he said. 'Maybe next time?' '*Si, la proxima vez*,' I agreed. A hug and a formal kiss.

In the taxi, while the others chattered, I reflected on the warmth of the tango communities here and in Cambridge. It would be good to be back.

Lesson notes

As we approach the end of the year, I'm drawn to that familiar two-way pull, the compulsion to look forward and to look back. 'This time last year...' we say, our instinct to measure the distance. For me, it's easier to think in terms of weight. I have the image of an old-fashioned balance – the kind still used, perhaps, in some pharmacological situations or for weighing silver or gold, with small circular pans – polished brass, in my mind – hanging from a pivoted central beam. In one pan the unknown quantity, in the other a known weight or mass, changing the latter until you achieve equilibrium, or thereabouts; fine-tuning can be done with a sliding bar, if there is one. The image, for me, comes complete with a memory of a school cloakroom, the rows of pegs outside the toilets where I used to sneak a quick fag during PE. I was one of a small gaggle of girls watching half-heartedly while our teacher demonstrated the process on a miniature set of scales. What were we doing in the cloakroom? Why such a small group? I think it must have been sixth form, and an enterprising English teacher (so now I know who) searching for a way to illustrate a point – Shylock's pound of flesh,[2] perhaps, or Hotspur's 'cavil on the ninth part of a hair'?[3] – by borrowing the scales from the lab next to the cloakroom. This time more than fifty years ago...

I arrive for my lesson, the first for a while, with flowers, a bargain two-for-£5 anemones from the market. We chat as John sweeps the floor. I've slept for four hours, which is becoming almost normal, so I'm beset by aching back and shoulders, and a creeping weariness – or is it misery? The sun is shining, though. We drink coffee. 'Life is good,' John says, broom in hand. Then we begin.

We work on disassociation, where we left off at the end of the last lesson. We practise the mid-torso twist, then the movement between a close and more open embrace, then *ochos* and *giros*. Now pace, particularly the first side step of the *giro*. In a way, this is reminiscent of those early days, when delay before a step was an issue. Now this is an easier thing to tackle, and I relish the feeling when it works. We speak about confidence and energy, stepping up to do more than just follow, to take 50 per cent of the responsibility – in effect, to dance. I mention two dancers whose positive stepping I admire. It is hard, I say, but I can do it. John nods. 'Yes, a challenge. I'm excited about these *giros*.' At once I'm snivelling, apologising that another sleep-light night has left me raw, as if I've lost a layer of skin.

The way time changes things… A month ago or so, one of our tango friends was celebrating the delights of a new direction in her work, an opportunity to work in the public sphere with experts in their field. Soon afterwards she and her husband learned of a large tumour in his chest. At last night's milonga she appeared dazed, and smaller somehow. She didn't talk much, but she hardly sat down. At the end of every set, another partner would emerge, hug her, open his arms for the embrace. As for me, almost a year ago, I thought I had problems with balance but that I might manage to build enough confidence to get by on the dance floor. I didn't see beyond the confines of my own limitations any more than Shylock did when he claimed his pound of flesh. You can have everything you ask for, he was told, but be warned: it takes almost nothing – the 'twentieth part of one poor scruple' – to tip the balance.

A scruple, apparently, was a tiny weight used by an apothecary, and the twentieth part of a scruple was a grain. And when you've imagined the smallness of a grain, think smaller. If the scale turns, Portia told Shylock, 'But in the estimation of a hair,' he will lose everything. I think of the lighter pan on the brass balance shooting up with the euphoria of my achievement, the sudden dip of the other that comes with middle-of-the-night despair.

I suppose the best thing, or one of the best, is finding out that you don't know everything you thought you did. Thank goodness for Ellie in this respect, always ready to remind us that this is a learning process for all three of us – 'organic' is her favourite term. So as well as working on holding my head up and feeling the floor, and pushing past what I can't do, I'm learning some late lessons about true friends and the support of a community.

The hour over, John puts a new saddle on my bike and pumps up my tyres. On balance, it's been a good year.

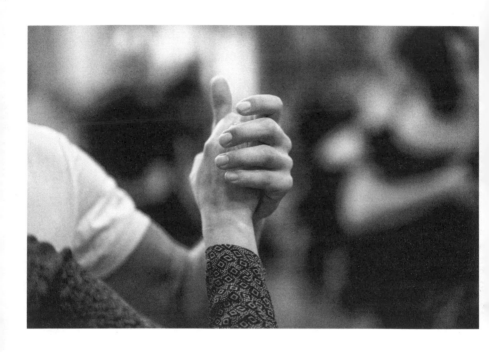

December:
The Dark Side

The song 'Button Up Your Overcoat', written in 1929 and memorably recorded by Helen Kane in the same year, offers an exhaustive list of precautions for a new lover (early nights, healthy eating, don't antagonise traffic cops, avoid stinging insects and strong liquor) because, the singer insists, you 'belong' to me.[1] Dictionary definitions of 'belong' often begin with 'to be rightly placed'. Additional meanings include 'to be a member of a group' and 'to have in one's possession'. I think of my friend Liz's reminder about children: contrary to how we feel about them, our children don't belong to us; rather, they are lent for a time. I suppose that is a truth, though a hard one to live with. Liz was the first person I visited with my tiny Jack in a pram shortly after we came out of hospital. I still have a book of hers, about Quakers, on a shelf somewhere – she was a Friend herself, as well as a friend to me. So I was shocked recently by the news of her death. Although she suffered from breast cancer several years ago, she had been well for some time, so her death was sudden, caused by a very aggressive form of leukaemia. When her older boy, Daniel, was seventeen, he also was diagnosed with leukaemia, after months of unidentified illness, at a time when the disease was both rare and usually regarded as incurable. He did recover, eventually. Later, Liz became my supervisor during my early days as a counsellor (I'd trained in an attempt to find an alternative to teaching but abandoned it when my marriage collapsed). I don't know quite where Liz belonged. Originally from the south of England, she remained rooted in rural north-east Cumbria while I moved south to Cambridge. We lost touch, crossing paths only occasionally. The last time I saw her, we exchanged phone numbers. And now another memory yabbers insistently in my ear. For a while, out of work and suddenly a single parent with a family to support, Liz cleaned our little house in Moat Street once a week. Her advice: polish your taps – a big return for a small outlay if you're pushed for time.

'Belonging' also seems to imply a situation where you feel comfortable, where you have a right to be. Of course, it's subjective: this sense that the place and its people are there to meet you. Unannounced, a memory from almost twenty years ago: as a teacher and alto saxophone player, I accompanied the school's dance band on the first leg of a transatlantic exchange. We arrived by coach in a remote corner of upstate New York early one evening, twenty-four hours later than expected. We were hot, dirty, tired, far from home. As we pulled into a car park, a smattering of figures shifted into a ragged line and moved towards us. The coach door opened. We dragged ourselves down the steps, shuffling on stiff legs. From somewhere in the centre of the line, a woman's voice (the adults were mostly women, I think; the youngsters, for the time being, hung back in a cartoon of cool) wavered the first notes of 'This Land Is Your Land'. Other voices joined hers. I think her arms were open – at least that is how I remember the moment: that beyond sentiment, a brief squirm at the cliché and a flicker of an echo of Woody Guthrie, here were arms and hearts ready to welcome us as we were, to a place where we already belonged. The car park moment held us for the coming weeks in a 'dry' town with a strongly evangelical Christian base, surrounded by small farms and bears in the woods. We swam in the pond. (When I returned with my son years later, he was terrified of the frogs and the oversized dragonflies.)

One of the challenges for the writer of what might be termed an 'illness narrative' can be the desire to be positive, rather than to moan. This is particularly so when the narrative takes on the shape of a quest, if not for a cure then at least for some less tangible benefit. In her discussion of the interpretation of patients' stories,[2] Professor Johanna Shapiro, Director of Medical Humanities and Arts at University of California Irvine, School of Medicine, suggests that the constraints of the narrative may lead the writer to present a view that even a 'devastating medical condition' is somehow for the best, making it difficult to express more negative emotions such as 'anger, despair, suffering, failure or protest'.[3] For me, there were times, naturally enough, when some, if not all, of these clamoured to be heard. While 'suffering' for me was generally limited to relatively minor annoyances – aches and pains, stiffness, insomnia, digestive uncertainty, fatigue – anger and the rest were always there, jostling just below the surface, looking for an opportunity to break through. Occasionally they managed it: frightening for me because they had a way of making it seem as if they were the 'real' story, and frightening for others, I imagine, for their suddenness and their venom. It was as if I'd been hijacked and was powerless to defend myself against these feelings or to protect those close to me. At times, I felt myself sucked into the silky waters of despair.

Writer John Burnside is familiar with the dark side, which makes the persistence of hope in his work especially valuable. A poem from his collection *Black Cat Bone* illustrates this well: 'Pieter Brueghel: Winter Landscape with Skaters and Bird Trap, 1565'. The painting on which the poem is based depicts what at first sight might be an idyllic winter scene of skaters who rediscover the innocent joy of childhood as they glide across the ice, although Burnside reminds us of the various hardships the skaters have left behind at home. For the artist, the precarious nature of our happiness is reflected in the bird trap in the foreground of the picture, the birds' obliviousness to the danger a mirror of our own unawareness of the risks we face. Burnside insists, though, that what matters is that a man may find himself.

> *gifted with the grace*
> *to skate for ever, slithering as he goes,*
> *but hazarding a guess that someone else*
> *is close beside him, other to his other.*[4]

Like the skaters on the ice, perhaps, in tango I was finding opportunities to live freely in the moment, in the confidence that I was not entirely alone.

Inevitably the gloom returned, set in like a spell of February cold, although gloom is the wrong word. This beast was an unlovely misshape of fury and despair that lurched persistently into my path. Whether I tried to step round it or kick it out of the way, or to look elsewhere, it was still there, shoving me off balance, snapping at my ankles. I found myself crying a lot — great snorting sobs that originated somewhere around the solar plexus and ripped up through my rib cage. It wasn't about anything in particular, although there was a smell of loneliness and failure about it, and terror. I was afraid that it wouldn't go away, that nothing — not tango, nor the love of friends, nor medicine, nor any amount of tap-polishing — would fix it. I was scared that this was early damage, never resolved; that there was a pattern of breaking things — friendships, relationships — before they broke me. I worried that this was the onset of dementia, and that these descents would become more precipitous. I couldn't see past it. If I held it inside, it acted like acid in my gut until it wouldn't be contained any longer. If I let it out, it smacked weakly against those who were close enough to touch. It was too feeble to cause much pain, but how long before the smart and the dreariness of the repeat caused those closest to me to move away? I knew there was nothing endearing about petulance or irrationality or despair.

One day I found myself on King's Parade, amongst the madness that is central Cambridge: students and tourists and kids, punt touts and beggars, cameras clicking, a dozen different languages, laughter, shorts and sandals, sunglasses and overcoats and umbrellas. The man in the bin played his guitar and sang, the centre of a shifting crowd of the incredulous and the idly curious. I sat on the wall just along from him, invisible. It was unusually warm for winter. I couldn't seem to move. I could think of nowhere to go, no one to call, no way to get past this moment, no possible future. I sat there for most of the day. Eventually, as afternoon threatened to become evening, I stepped back from the brink and made two phone calls: first, to the doctor for an appointment and secondly to my son, who came and sat with me. At last, just before it got dark, we walked home.

At the very end of the year I saw for the second time the lovely French film *The Artist*, a homage to the era of the silent movie. Afterwards we walked back through a city almost silenced by snow. The following morning the promised four inches blanketed cars and pavements. I welcomed the prospect of an enforced withdrawal, feeling too mean and difficult for company, finding the written word kinder. I searched for my school copy of T. S. Eliot's *Selected Poems*, but it seemed to have been lost in the move. 'These fragments I have shored against my ruins'[5] was the line I needed, from 'The Waste Land'. I thought about the muddy waters of the rivers – various rivers – flowing through that poem and, elsewhere, of Prufrock's grim recognition that we can linger in the sea caverns with the mermaids only for so long, until 'human voices wake us, and we drown'.[6] I searched the internet poetry archive and listened to Stevie Smith introducing and then reading her poem 'Not Waving But Drowning'.[7] I thought of oily waters stroking a shoulder. I returned to Julian Barnes's *The Sense of an Ending*:

> I thought – at some level of my being, I actually thought – that I could go back to the beginning and change things. That I could make the blood flow backwards.[8]

In *The Artist*, the erstwhile star of the silent screen retreats until he sits with an empty glass on a chair in a room empty of everything except the reels of film that represent his entire working life. In a frenzy – indulgent, impotent, ridiculous, as all such frenzies are – he sets about destroying them, ripping open cans, tearing at spools of film, eventually setting light to the pile. At the moment when all is sure to be lost, as flames and smoke threaten to overcome him, he clutches to his chest one canister. At times such as these, what else is there to do but take hold of the broken pieces and hold them close?

If you haven't seen the film yet, I'm sure it won't spoil it for you to know that there is a happy ending – although not one either protagonist would have wished for, perhaps.

Lesson notes

It's been roughly a year since that first lesson, when I met Kate off the train (or forgot to, as she points out!) and was scratching my head about her wobbly right arm and how to tackle it. In that time we have seen wonderful progress in her ability to move gracefully and confidently, but of course things can't continue at the same rate...

— John

So, we've been dancing together a year, almost exactly, you say. We begin with a check on the confidence factor of following a more subtle lead – back, side, forward. It feels good. I think about posture, concentrate on holding up the upper body and chest, core engaged but shoulders relaxed, while keeping a sense that the feet are rooted in the floor. My body stretches along its axis, along the length of the spine and from the ball of the foot to the crown of the head. The front of my body meets yours, listens for your intention, your breathing, the clench and release of muscle.

I feel a wash of relief: this tango thing does still work. In bleak recent weeks, near-overwhelmed by exhaustion and struggling with the black hole of depression that yawns in front of me, I have been frightened that the benefits have weakened as my tolerance of them has increased. Or is it simply that the disease has stepped up its progress? I try to explain, again, the necessity for me of keeping going, as well as the difficulties. For example, in order to get to the point on a Tuesday night where several hours of tango will replace fatigue with energy and despair with optimism, I have first to get past the fatigue and despair sufficiently just to arrive at the milonga. Often, lately, the getting past has seemed too difficult.

Maybe we need to push you harder, you say. We dance a few songs in an open embrace, where there is less support, simply for the challenge. We are both surprised, I think, by how well I cope. We squabble a little over *ganchos* and *barridas*, focusing on the axis rather than the quality of the figure. We are distracted briefly by the absence, or not, of the second of the two notes at the end of a song (the 'chan chan'). You replay the last few bars and yes, it is there, so quiet that it almost isn't there at all. Sol *doh*, you say.

We are deep in Pugliese territory now, but the familiar is laced with the new. I try to explain something of my anxiety: that we are past the 'special project' stage, the mutual excitement of discovery, as other new ventures push their way forward. Now it's the hard graft, you say. We talk over ways we can introduce more challenge, find a way of moving on. We finish with 'Nochero Soy', an established favourite now, and then one more.

The following morning at five o'clock, I give up all pretence of sleep. My arms and legs ache, and I'm oppressed by the mountain of things I have to do against the backdrop of another wakeful night. I think back over yesterday's lesson – calm, reflective, full of hope – and over the year of lessons.

Last week I arrived in a dismal fury, sobbed my way through a tangle of misery and frustration while you sat next to me, nodded, laughed sometimes, fastened my shoes. We managed maybe half an hour of tango while I snuffled with the aftershock. I've never danced with someone who's crying before, you said. For some reason I remember the summer's evening we met on Mill Road for a curry, and then another memory: the story of the Tibetan prayer flags spread round the garden you had left behind. My right shoulder jumps and squirms. So much of what happens is beyond our control. But this – this precious thing, the learning and friendship, strength and safety; I tried to explain yesterday, again, how important these have been for me. You listen and nod, as if you are hearing this for the first time. Sometimes I turn up with flowers. If you're too busy to notice me, I'm prone to squally protest. Yesterday I forgot to pay you for the lesson. None of this matters. I don't have to explain: you know. I imagine a stone on the palm of my hand, smooth, unmoving. I close my fingers over it. In noise or danger, in the dark, I can keep it safe. It will still be there.

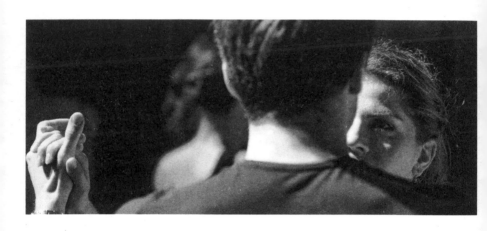

Epilogue

Initially, Kate was looking for an 'expert', keen for my involvement because of my tango experience and my psychology background. I realised quite quickly that working with Kate on this project demanded a different approach. My role became more like holding a torch so we could check out the routes together, rather than providing a map or offering directions. There was no fixed destination, but a shared belief that reflection on experience leads to learning.

— Ellie

It's more than eight years since I stepped off the train for that first lesson with John and, inevitably, much has changed. Ellie's hands soon became too full for torch-holding, with a house move then renovation, and the birth of one then a second daughter. John is rarely available for private lessons these days, a new job not the least of other demands on his time. In fact, by the end of that first year, the alliance of the 'Three Musketeers' – as Ellie had christened us – was already beginning to feel shaky. My dark moods grew darker and more frequent. As I found things more difficult, I needed more help. Rather like the greedy young blackbird that stands outside my window most mornings, mouth open, waiting for it to be filled, however much went in, I was still hungry. At some point I must have understood, as the blackbird no doubt will, that what others could give would never be enough and that it was time I sought out my own nourishment.

One change happened, eventually, in response to the English National Ballet's Dance for Parkinson's programme.[1] When I first heard of it, some years after its 2008 launch, my gut reaction was hostile. The BBC news video showed part of a class of forty adults with Parkinson's and their carers. The class was based on *The Nutcracker*, the group divided into mice and soldiers. As I watched, I felt – what? Not just put off, but unaccountably angry. The clip ended with their final bow: 'Everybody join hands together.' My response? I won't. I wouldn't be herded into a hall like that and have therapy 'done' to me. I didn't want to be told whether I was a mouse or a soldier. And I certainly didn't want to be defined by my Parkinson's.

However, when a friend passed on to me an invitation to sign up for a Dance for Parkinson's Professional Development Weekend for dance artists and teachers, run by English National Ballet at Dance East in Ipswich, I was intrigued. It was stretching a point – I was hardly a dance professional – but at this stage John, Ellie and I were still hoping to offer supported tango tuition in mainstream classes in Cambridge for people with Parkinson's, so I signed up and went along. The weekend began with introductions. When it came to my turn, stupidly, on the spur of the moment, I ducked out of the opportunity to confess that I had a foot in both camps, anxious that, if they knew, they would send me home. So I spent the rest of the weekend trying to conceal my Parkinson's. That aside, by the end of the first morning I was a convert, impressed by the methodical and sensitive way in which the classes moved from one stage to the next, each one targeting a particular aspect of the condition, yet managing throughout to keep the emphasis on dance rather than disease. I came clean immediately afterwards – in any case, I now wanted to join the Ipswich group as a participant.

I took part in all the next term's classes – *The Nutcracker* again – and learned so much. First, of course no one wants to be defined by the disease – why did I imagine I would be alone in that? But perhaps acceptance could help me to become less judgemental towards illness and disability, my own and others'? Second, how much I enjoyed the chance to practise ballet! The voice work, an integral part of each class, focusing on confidence and volume in speech and singing, was of particular benefit to me; and, increasingly, what a pleasure and a privilege it was to be part of that group, and to be accepted in my entirety. What was it the lawyer Alfieri said of Eddie in Arthur Miller's *A View from the Bridge*? He loved him more than all his more sensible clients because he allowed himself to be 'wholly known'.[2] Here was an environment in which I really didn't have to hide anything. Finally, that joining-hands moment at the end of each class: it seemed that what we had in common created a powerful emotional bond and I never got through it entirely dry-eyed.

The following summer, a bonus: an opportunity to join a class in Leicester run by David Leventhal, programme director and founding teacher of the Mark Morris Dance Group's Dance for PD programme. Given my love of the company's work, David Leventhal was already something of a hero. More than this, he seemed to understand intuitvely what it feels like to live with Parkinson's and how liberating dance can be:

> Dance requires mind and imagination, focus and physicality. So does living with Parkinson's. It's grace that's hard won… Dance gives people an opportunity to experience what it's like to move with grace and to move with power and to move with passion…[3]

The Leicester class was based on *West Side Story*. I don't recall now if I was a Shark or a Jet, only how exciting it was to share a dance space with David, to experience at first hand his creative energy, his belief in the transformative power of dance and the joy that comes from being part of a community of dancers.

Still, the Parkinson's was taking its course, frustratingly unpredictable in its apparently random 'on' and 'off' states, progressing at its own pace, although I'm sure its advance was hampered by the dancing and further delayed by regular yoga, swimming, walking, and a little two-wheeled wobbling. It certainly became more noticeable, though, the dyskinesias – those involuntary wrigglings and writhings which often accompany the condition – rattling round my body sometimes like a bucketful of frogs, until I appeared quite drunk. In a pub one Saturday evening, a lady who'd evidently had a few herself tried to persuade me to try strawberry cider 'although you look like you've been rocking a bit already'. I never found a satisfactory reaction to comments like these – probably coolest to say I'd been at the champagne and leave a little envy in my wake?

In October 2017 I was offered a solution of sorts in the shape of deep brain stimulation, a surgical procedure involving the insertion of electrodes into the brain, controlled by a device beneath the skin of the chest. The procedure has more than lived up to its reputation as a life-changer: the dyskinesias are gone, along with the rigidity and most of the tremor. The surgeon's insistence on a full head shave also left me with a new look, which I decided to keep. On the minus side, my balance has been less good, with inevitable repercussions on the dance floor.

Still, tango remains the bedrock of my treatment, a fundamental part of my health and well-being, the mainstay of my social life, a source of support and a regular opportunity for delight, although it's rarely plain sailing. Like any ageing *tanguera*, at times I find myself overlooked in favour of younger, prettier, better dancers. As any tango dancer will tell you, there are those who used to dance with me and no longer do, and others who never have and never will. Like any dancer worth her salt, I strive to be better. I'm aware of a tension in Cambridge Tango between aspiration – naturally it wants to build its reputation for excellence – and inclusion. Much of the time it manages to do both. Meanwhile, there are times when I have to settle for the cakes and ale version, helping to organise and run events, baking for special occasions, putting on a brave face when I find myself in a conversation about classes for advanced dancers or the next trip abroad for a tango marathon, opportunities now out of reach for me.

But on the whole, tango is wonderful. I know that stepping onto the dance floor is an opportunity for transformation. With some partners, I can take pleasure in being more adventurous as we respond to the music. A handful of particular leaders have made this possible for me, keeping me in their sights, pushing the boundaries of what we can do together and enjoying, even relishing, the results. One friend turns up at my house every week for a one-to-one practice session. I have also begun to enjoy the role of the tango DJ. The responsibility for choosing and delivering the music for three and a half hours of dancing can be nerve-wracking, but it's also exciting and I hope will offer a way of continuing to be part of the tango community when taking to the dance floor is no longer an option.

On days when I simply can't get any part of me to behave, I remember Julian. He was from the Newcastle area although I first met him at Salon Canning in Buenos Aires, by which time he was already living with a terminal illness. I saw him again in Argentina a couple of years later, as he disappeared into an epic storm with Francesca in search of a dance class. Apparently they ended up sitting on the pavement in a red-light district drinking Quilmes at five o'clock in the morning. The next time I saw him was the last, at a tea dance in the Tithe Barn in Carlisle. We spoke briefly, and didn't dance together. He died some years ago now, leaving these instructions for his funeral:

> No scruffy people allowed into the service. Anyone not crying to get a Chinese burn to help them to do so.

Francesca tells me she heard from Julian shortly before his death; he was looking forward to dancing with her at the next milonga, 'though I probably won't be able to manage a whole song'. Francesca replied something along the lines of, 'Well, your singing was never up to much anyway.' She told me he danced his last dances with his oxygen tank on his back.

His death takes me to others we have lost whose lives provide inspiration for the living. 'Tango Dave', notable for his waxed moustache and his invariable dress shirt and shorts, died recently at the age of fifty-one. A funeral Mass in Little St Mary's on Valentine's Day was followed by a suitably lavish celebration at the University Social Club. Most recently Gerry, tireless mainstay of milongas and tea dances, always there for running repairs, shifting chairs, serving tea and coffee, and washing up (he was also a lovely if unassuming dancer) passed away in hospital. My extraordinary friend Liz (another Liz) died suddenly following a long illness, after spending Christmas with her family. She was full of plans for more travel, more paintings, more projects. Her written commentary on her artwork *This Work Is Not Finished* might have been a statement of faith.

My dad left us one spring. He hung on through my birthday until the following morning, when he gave Jack and me cards that he had written. The handwriting is heartbreakingly cramped and wandering, almost entirely illegible. He slept for much of the rest of the day. In the night, he called for his father, seemed to see us, then turned away, curled on his side. The gaps between breaths grew longer, until eventually they stopped. I read Philip Larkin's 'The Trees' at his funeral. My mum outlived him by fourteen years, her last refrain, 'I'm very lucky, aren't I?' One late pleasure was a day in Cambridge's Botanic Garden when she allowed herself to be pushed along in a wheelchair as John took photos.

So – there is John, still, of course. While the private lessons have gone, he is still very much present. Our friendship has had some bumpy patches, and I remember a couple of spectacular shouting matches. But the intensity of those early days has settled into something more durable as I've become more stable and less demanding. When we dance, as we still do sometimes, he is both empathetic and creative, and he continues to be a patient, loyal and generous friend. There is often room for laughter. I feel immensely grateful.

As for the future: who knows? Shockwaves from the wider world – political, environmental – clamour for our attention. My own upheavals as I moved house yet again were put into perspective by the massive refugee crisis. Even the tango world had to respond and we held a tea dance in support of Médecins Sans Frontières. More recently, there is the madness that is Brexit. In terms of our smaller futures, too, we can never know what is coming next.

In November 2011, members of the Brooklyn Dance for Parkinson's class found themselves at the centre of David Iverson's documentary film, *Capturing Grace* (2014), about their preparations for a stage performance. A comment from Cyndy, one of the dancers, has stayed with me:

> When you think that your life is not going to hold
> any more surprises, here comes this wonderful gift.[4]

Tango reminds us that uncertainty can be something to cherish. Perhaps I can learn to view Parkinson's in a similar light, savouring its unpredictability, living more fully in the present moment, open to whatever possibilities may unfold.

Appendix
Touch: A Short Story

tango *syncopated ballroom dance, 1913, from Argentine Sp. tango, originally the name of an African-American drum dance, probably from a Niger-Congo language (cf. Ibibio tamgu 'to dance'). Phrase* it takes two to tango *was a song title from 1952* [1]

[*Latin:* verb present active *tangō*, present infinitive <u>*tangere*</u>, perfect active <u>*tetigī*</u>, supine <u>*tāctum*</u>, <u>transitive</u> *I* <u>touch, grasp</u>]

As soon as it was over she pulled on her boots, kissed him twice in the usual way and left, closing the door behind her. Birds chattered from the top of the tree at the end of the garden. She bumped down the steps, crunched across the gravel and round the corner, then through the gate by the railway line, the grace of the last sixty minutes or so already gone. Only the grace, though: she felt still the charge, the pulse, the ripple and twist of sensation as the ordinariness of the tiny station clattered around her. Busier today: two street drinkers (this was how she thought of them) on the first seat, one male and a younger female, cans in hand, loud but not too quarrelsome; a clutch of kids (youths, her mother would say), the woman in the red coat pushing a bike, as always, a man with a suitcase on wheels. 12:08 the orange letters on the electronic board but the train was late – even a couple of minutes' delay would mean the meeting would have started by the time she got there. She considered the perfect moment to reach the platform. 'Don't run,' he'd said the first time. 'You're way too early.' He was right, of course; years as a commuter, he explained later, gave him a perfect sense of the six minutes it took from… She couldn't recall the names. He laughed at her anxious clock-checking, though not unkindly. 'I think you're getting the hang of it,' he said after the second session. The train, he meant. 12:11, so perhaps three minutes to arrive, collect and be ready – if the train was on time. She smiled at the thought of the clocks in the house – four at least, she had seen – all at different times, one stopped at 11:25 – as if the hour might last for ever.

Dust on her sleeve; another's breath on the back of her neck as they waited for the doors to open – she, who minutes before had worn him like a second skin, shrank from the contact. As the train pulled away she closed her eyes and yielded to the rise and fall of sound and movement that she carried in her core still, allowing it to flood her with its sweet, insidious warmth, right to her toenails, the backs of her knees. She felt for the long fingers twined through hers; the strength of his arm on her back –

released for a second, and then a firmer embrace; the fluttery moment before her cheek finds its place beneath his chin. She feels herself unfurl, a flower opening in the warmth of the sun, her shadows exposed to the light, as beautiful and as unremarkable as the petals of a daisy. She waits, then shifts her head an inch until she can feel his heart beating; or perhaps it is the echo of her own heart. She listens, looks for his intention. They breathe. When he moves, she will move with him entirely, precisely, so that they move as one body, one being.

Is it wrong to be so preoccupied with the body? It is a legacy of her childhood; that an interest in the physical comes with its own burden of guilt. Even so, she won't be deterred: she considers the work of muscle clenching, relaxing; the fine strength of bone; the kind warmth of flesh; the quiet journey of the breath, the give and take of the lungs. She recalls the dip of his head, the eyebrow raised above closed eyes at a certain cadence. She relishes the symmetry of her response – Narcissus in his pool: in the mirror of his loveliness she becomes lovely, savouring the delicious miracle that allows her to experience poise as if she were whole again. 'I need you to be more compliant,' he said. They laughed, although beneath the irony lay a truth: these moments revolved precisely around the spot where push meets resistance, the place between stop and surrender.

It is the perfect gift: unexpected, undeserved, unsolicited, unstinting; a giving that understands exactly what the receiver wishes and, beyond awareness, needs. Like the party game, beneath each layer there is more, the end still not in sight. Weak with gratitude, fierce with devotion, like a cat at the banister, fickle and furious, she demands attention as soon as he is near. Her jealous claws flex. She will leave a sparrow at his door, the splintered bones hidden under the sheen of feathers. Perhaps she will keep a paw on the folded wing until he appears.

In fact, the next day begins in non-predatory fashion, with piano music, the cool notes of Eric Satie dripping into the early light. She remembers another morning: Mozart bubbling through the room at the front of the house, where he stood with his back to her at the window, scanning the skies. And piano again, but this time silenced; she watches from the bus window as a man about her own age tips a quantity of rum into half a plastic bottle of Coke, tastes the mix and then, tucking it in his pocket, runs his fingers over invisible keys in expansive runs and flourishes while he harangues the queue. She sees them turn away one by one, indifference, boredom, embarrassment prevailing; only one, older, lady steps towards him, her mouth working, one arm raised. 'Gave him a piece of my mind,' she imagines the woman reporting back later. The voice becomes a tune in her head which is taken up by the strings and then melts into the raw longing of the bandoneon, its lascivious tongue licking the line from her navel to her chin, redolent with yearning, slick with satisfaction.

Of course, perfection, like consummation, is transitory. In time – who knows how much time? – the disease will take a stronger hold, rough hands gripping her limbs, pinning her heavy and stupid in the place she doesn't wish to be – clumsy, fumbling, out of kilter; or will send her hands skittering, tipping a full glass across white linen. She will be known by the shuffle in her step, the tremor of a hand. Perhaps her face will droop or her speech slur. She avoids the thought of worse indignities. For now, she will plunder whatever satisfaction she can find, plunging greedy hands into the barrel, grabbing joy before it slithers beyond her grasp and trapping it, squeezing it tight in closed fists, never letting go. 'Trust me,' people say. She would trust him with her life, stretched out patient on the tracks, safe in the knowledge that he will be there in time to pluck her from disaster. 'I feel you are on my side,' she said to him once. 'I am on your side,' he said.

Today there is a crowd on the platform: green waterproofs, tripods and cameras. Binoculars point to a rash of birds, starling-sized, at the top of a bush covered in berries scarlet as new blood: an irruption of waxwings, arrived from Scandinavia. Delight fizzes and crackles around the watching heads. The train is late again. She looks obediently through a telescope. Instead of the nondescript brown shape she expects, there is a plump, indignant creature, plumage flushed with pink, a crest swept back as if by a sudden gust; flamboyant, uncompromising, gorgeous. The wing is flashed with yellow, red and white.

On the train, lingering in the warmth of the close embrace, she looks upwards through the smear of the window. Even with the naked eye she can see the livid splash of the wing bars, a head turned unflinching into the wind, the blush of the fruits, a tracery of twigs against an impossibly blue sky.

Appendix II
Tremulous

For Kate

Inadvertent, the gift
That presses out of you,
To modulate and soon to soothe
My own composure
Whereupon all pomp of posture
Falls away.
Only the essence of the dance,
The shape of breath that you impose
Embellished by its mystery
Remains.
The small spectacle of our passing
And me
No longer tremulous.

[Ray Harper Poems, 2012]

Glossary

amor — love

bandoneon — the accordion-like instrument that is the sound and soul of tango

bandoneonista — bandoneon player

barrida — a tango move where a dancer uses a foot to sweep the partner's free foot along the floor

barrio — neighbourhood

boina — beret, cap

boleo — a figure where the leader changes direction, causing the follower's leg to swing out along the floor (from *bolear* — to throw)

buen viaje — have a good trip

cabeceo — a nod: the unspoken invitation to dance

candombe — drumming and dance from Africa via Uruguay, and an essential feature of street life in San Telmo, the oldest *barrio* in Buenos Aires

capitán — captain

cara fea — literally 'ugly face', the cold stare adopted by some early *tangueros*

chacarera – a folk dance which interrupts every milonga in
   Buenos Aires

chicas – girls

conventillo – a tenement block, home to poor immigrant
   families in early twentieth-century Buenos Aires

corazón – heart

emancipación – emancipation, but also the name of a
   wonderfully edgy tango recorded by Osvaldo Pugliese's
   orchestra in 1955

empanada – a pasty traditionally filled with beef, though
   alternatives – even vegetarian – are becoming more
   widespread; available at most *milongas*

estribillista – a singer of refrains

estudio de danzas – dance studio

farol – lamp post, but also the name of a tango made
   famous by Osvaldo Pugliese's orchestra, with lyrics by
   poet Homero Expósito

flojo/a – loose

gancho – literally 'hook'; a figure where a dancer hooks
   a leg round the partner's leg in a quick flick; exciting
   in performance but can be dangerous, and therefore
   frowned on in social tango

giro – literally 'turn'; a figure where one dancer (usually
   the follower) walks around the partner (from *girar* – to
   turn)

hola/buenos noches/que tal? – hello/good evening/how are
   you?

la próxima vez – the next time

lo siento – I'm sorry

Lunfardo – Buenos Aires slang, often used in early tango lyrics

manos – hands

mariposa – butterfly, and the name of a 1923 tango, with several recordings including one by Osvaldo Pugliese's orchestra

milonga – a dance hall and, by extension, the event held there. Also a specific style of music and dance related to tango, but usually faster

milonguero – a dancer at milongas, often an older dancer with years of expertise; by extension, *milonguero*-style is used to describe a traditional style of tango, danced in close embrace

molinete – literally 'windmill', an alternative name for the *giro*

muerte – death

nada – nothing, and the name of a 1944 tango recorded by many orchestras

Niebla del Riachuelo – literally 'Fog on the Riachuelo' (a little river, here specifically the Matanza River), and the name of a tango recorded by various orchestras, including a 1937 version by Osvaldo Fresedo's orchestra, with *estribillista* Roberto Ray

noche – night

nunca mas – never again

oblivión – oblivion, but also the name of a haunting tango by Astor Piazzolla that has featured in several films *ocho* – a figure-of-eight move where the leader directs the follower in alternating turning steps

ojos – eyes

orquesta – orchestra

práctica – practice

porteño – someone from the 'port', i.e. in Buenos Aires, a local

Quilmes – our favourite beer in Buenos Aires

recuerdo – a memory, souvenir (from *recordar* – to remember)

sacada – literally 'displacement'; a movement in which one dancer deliberately invades the partner's floor space

soledad – loneliness

El Subte – the Buenos Aires metro

sentada – a 'sitting' or 'seated' figure, where a follower appears to sit on the leader's thigh, sometimes used as an embellishment at the end of a dance

tanda – a set of three or four songs; etiquette suggests that you dance the full set with the same partner

tango nuevo – literally 'new tango', referring to developments in the style of dance characterised by a more elastic embrace and innovation

tanguero/a – a tango dancer

traspié – literally 'a stumble', and a quick step where a dancer begins to change weight and then immediately retreats to the original position

tres esquinas – literally 'three corners', and the name of a tango recorded by Ángel D'Agostino and Ángel Vargas in 1941

Una pregunta: hay cambio? – One question: do you have change?

vals – a tango in waltz-time

vida – life

volcada – a movement typical of *tango nuevo* where the follower is out of axis and the dancers are leaning towards each other (from *volcar* – to overturn)

volver – literally 'to return', and the name of a famous 1935 tango by Carlos Gardel

vuelvo al sur – I'm going back to the south, and the title of a 1988 tango by Astor Piazzolla

Credits

Image Credits

Bibliography

Allen, J. L., McKay, J. L. et al., 'Increased neuromuscular consistency in gait and balance after partnered dance-based rehabilitation in Parkinson's disease', *Journal of Neurophysiology* 118, July 2017, pp. 363–73

Armitage, Simon, *Book of Matches*, Faber & Faber, London, 1993

Barnes, Julian, *The Sense of an Ending*, Jonathan Cape, London, 2011

Blonder, L. X., Slevin, J. T., 'Emotional Dysfunction in Parkinson's Disease', *Behavioural Neurology* 24 (3), 2011

Bognar, S., DeFaria, A. M., et al., 'More than just dancing: experiences of people with Parkinson's disease in a therapeutic dance program', *Disability and Rehabilitation*, 39(11), June 2017

Burnside, John, *Black Cat Bone*, Jonathan Cape, London, 2011

Burnside, John, *Waking Up in Toytown*, Vintage, London, 2010

Canning, C. G., Ada, L., Woodhouse, E., 'Multiple-task walking training in people with mild to moderate

Parkinson's disease: a pilot study', *Clinical Rehabilitation* 22(3), March 2008

Connatty J., McKenny, E., Swindlehurst, K., 'Tango and Parkinson's: the view from the dance floor', *Animated*, Winter 2013. Also available at www.communitydance. org.uk/DB/animated-library/tango-and-parkinsons-the-view-from-the-dance-floor

Davis, Kathy, *Dancing Tango: Passionate Encounters in a Globalizing World*, New York and London, New York University Press, 2015

Denniston, Christine, *The Meaning of Tango: The Story of the Argentinian Dance*, Portico, London, 2007

Duff, J., Gillespie, A., Fogg, A., 'Making it happen', *Animated*, Autumn 2011. Also available at www.communitydance. org.uk/DB/animated-library/making-it-happen

Eliot, T. S., *Selected Poems*, Faber & Faber, London, 1964

Fox, Michael J., *Lucky Man*, Hyperion, Westport, 2002

Gerecke, K., Jiao, Y. et al., 'Exercise protects against MPTP-induced neurotoxicity in mice', *Brain Research*, 1341, June 2010

Grealy, Lucy, *Autobiography of a Face*, Methuen, London, 2004

Hackney, M. E., Earhart, G. M., 'Effects of dance on movement control in Parkinson's disease: a comparison of Argentine tango and American ballroom', *Journal of Rehabilitation Medicine*, 41(6), May 2009

Hackney, M. E., Earhart, G. M., 'Recommendations for implementing tango classes for persons with Parkinson disease', *American Journal of Dance Therapy* 32, 2010

Hackney, M. E., Kantorovich, S. et al., 'Effects of tango on functional mobility in Parkinson's disease: a preliminary study', *Journal of Neurologic Physical Therapy* 31, 2007

Hughes, J. R., Bowes, S. G. et al., 'Parkinsonian abnormality of foot strike: a phenomenon of ageing and/or one responsive to levodopa therapy?' *British Journal of Clinical Pharmacology* 29, 1990

Hustvedt, Siri, *The Shaking Woman or A History of My Nerves*, Sceptre, London, 2010

Iverson, David, *Capturing Grace,* Kikim Media, 2014

Jekka, J. J., 'Light touch contact as a balance aid', *Physical Therapy* 77, 1997

Jones, Lloyd, *Here at the End of the World We Learn to Dance*, John Murray, London, 2008

Kassabova, Kapka, *Twelve Minutes of Love: A Tango Story*, Portobello Books, London, 2011

McGill, A., Houston, S., Lee, R. Y., 'Dance for Parkinson's: A new framework for research on its physical, mental, emotional and social benefits', *Complementary Therapies in Medicine* 22, 2014

McNeely, M. E., Mai, M. M. et al., 'Differential effects of tango versus Dance for PD in Parkinson's disease', *Frontiers in Aging Neuroscience* 7, 2015

Pethybridge, Ruth, *Into your Arms*, Film Oxford, 2010

Petzinger, G. M., Fisher, B. E. et al., 'Enhancing neuroplasticity in the basal ganglia: the role of exercise in Parkinson's disease', *Movement Disorders* 25, 2010.

Petzinger, G. M., Walsh, J. P. et al., 'Effects of treadmill exercise on dopaminergic transmission in the 1-methyl 4-phenyl-1,2,3,6-tetrahydropyridine-lesioned mouse model of basal ganglia injury', *The Journal of Neuroscience* 27 (20), 2007

Rocha, P. A., Slade, S. C. et al., 'Dance is more than therapy: qualitative analysis on therapeutic dancing classes for Parkinson's', *Complementary Therapies in Medicine* 34, 2017

Rogers, Carl, *On Becoming a Person: A Therapist's View of Psychotherapy*, Constable, London, 1961

Rogers, Carl, 'The Foundations of the Person-Centred Approach', *Education*, 100(2), Winter 1979, p. 98. Also available at www.elementsuk.com/libraryofarticles/foundations.pdf

Sacks, Oliver, *Musicophilia: Tales of Music and the Brain*, Picador, London, 2007

Savigliano, Marta, E., *Tango and the Political Economy of Passion*. Boulder, Colorado, 1995

Shapiro, Johanna, 'Illness narratives: reliability, authenticity and the empathic witness', *Medical Humanities*, 37, 2011

Taylor, Jonathan, *Take Me Home: Parkinson's, My Father, Myself*, Granta, London, 2007

Taylor, Julie, *Paper Tangos*, Duke University Press, Durham, Carolina, 1998

Thompson, Robert Farris, *Tango: The Art History of Love*, Vintage, London, 2006

Treitman, Helaine, *The Embrace of Aging*, now available as part of the series, *The Embrace Of*, Visionalist Entertainment

Productions, Michigan, 2017, https://theembraceofseries. vhx.tv/

de Waal, Edmund, *The Hare with Amber Eyes: A Hidden Inheritance*, Chatto and Windus, London, 2010

Woolf, Virginia, *A Room of One's Own*, Hogarth Press, London, 1928

Zigmond, M. J., Cameron, J. L., Hoffer, B. J. et al 'Neurorestoration by physical exercise: moving forward', *Parkinsonism and related disorders* 18, 2012

'Monkeys with Parkinson's disease benefit from human stem cells', *Science Daily*, August 30, 2017

'Connection between healthy ageing and neurodegenerative disorders', CORDIS EU research results, 2017, cordis. europa.eu/news/rcn/33891

Notes

INTRODUCTION
1 John Connatty, Ellie McKenny, Kate Swindlehurst, 'Tango and Parkinson's: The view from the dance floor', *Animated*, Winter 2013, pp. 16–18.
2 A. McGill, S. Houston, R.Y. Lee, 'Dance for Parkinson's: A new framework for research on its physical, mental, emotional and social benefits', *Complementary Therapies in Medicine*, 22(3), June 2014, pp. 426-32; see also P. Rocha, S.C. Slade, J. McClelland et al., 'Dance is more than therapy: qualitative analysis on therapeutic dancing classes for Parkinson's', *Complementary Therapies in Medicine*, 34, October 2017, pp. 1-9.

ONE: JANUARY
1 Michael J. Fox, *Lucky Man*, Hyperion, Westport, 2002, p. 293.

TWO: FEBRUARY
1 For current statistics see www.parkinsons.org.uk; www.parkinson.org
2 'Monkeys with Parkinson's disease benefit from human stem cells', *Science Daily*, 30 August 2017.
3 K. M. Gerecke, J. Yiao, A. Pani, 'Exercise protects against MPTP-induced neurotoxicity in mice', *Brain Research*, 1341, June 2010, pp. 72–83; M. J. Zigmond, Cameron, J. L., Hoffer, B. J. et al., 'Neurorestoration by physical exercise: moving forward', *Parkinsonism and Related Disorders*, 18 January 2012, pp. 147–50.
4 G. M. Petzinger, J. P. Walsh, G. Akopian et al., 'Effects of treadmill exercise on dopaminergic transmission in the 1-methyl-4-phenyl-1, 2, 3, 6-tetrahydropyridine-lesioned mouse model of basal ganglia injury', *The Journal of Neuroscience*, 27, May 2007, pp. 5291–300.
5 G.M. Petzinger, B. E. Fisher, J. E.Van Leeuwen et al., 'Enhancing neuroplasticity in the basal ganglia: the role of exercise in Parkinson's disease', *Movement Disorders*, 25, 2010, pp. 141–5.
6 M. E. Hackney, S. Kantorovich, R. Levin et al., 'Effects of tango on functional mobility in Parkinson's disease: a preliminary study', *Journal of Neurologic Physical Therapy*, 31, December 2007, pp. 173-9.
7 M. E. Hackney, G. M. Earhart, 'Effects of dance on movement control in Parkinson's disease: a comparison of Argentine tango and American

ballroom', *Journal of Rehabilitation Medicine* 41, May 2009, pp. 475–81; see also M. E. McNeely et al., 'Differential effects of tango versus dance for PD in Parkinson's disease', *Frontiers in Aging Neuroscience*, 7, December 2015, p. 239.

8 Madeleine Hackney (nominee for Groundbreaker of the Year Award for using the tango to treat mobility problems), *Atlanta*, Michele Cohen Marill, September 2016, http://www.atlantamagazine.com/groundbreakers-2016/madeleine-hackney/, see also Manatee Educational Television METV (2018); *Neuro Challlenge Session 4 Dance Therapies*, available at www.youtube.com/watch?v=4N2q1bXiTUs (accessed 3 June 2019); Dr Madeleine Hackney (2019), *Dancers of New York*, 28 November 2017, available at www.facebook.com/dancersofny/photos/rpp.528188157323490/1029035653905402/?type=3&theater (accessed 3 June 2019)

9 J. L. Allen, J. L. McKay, A. Sawers, M. E. Hackney, L. H. Ting, 'Increased neuromuscular consistency in gait and balance after partnered dance-based rehabilitation in Parkinson's disease', *Journal of Neurophysiology* 118, July 2017, pp. 363–73.

10 C. R. Rogers, *On Becoming a Person: a Therapist's View of Psychotherapy*, Constable, London, 1961, pp. 283–4.

11 C. R. Rogers, 'The actualizing tendency in relation to "motives" and to consciousness', in Marshall Jones (ed.), *Nebraska Symposium on Motivation*, Univ. of Nebraska Press, 1963, pp. 1–24. [an accessible later version 'The Foundations of the Person-Centred Approach', 1979, at http://www.elementsuk.com/libraryofarticles/foundations.pdf, s.v. 'actualizing tendency'.]

THREE: MARCH

1 Christine Denniston, *The Meaning of Tango: The Story of the Argentinian Dance*, Portico, London, 2007, p. 6.

2 Ibid. p. 20.

3 Simon Collier, Artemis Cooper, Maria Susan Azzi et al., *Tango! The Dance, the Song, the Story*, Thames & Hudson, London, 1995, p. 182.

4 Ibid p. 155.

5 Robert Farris Thompson, *Tango: The Art History of Love*, Vintage, London, 2006, p. 28.

6 Denniston, *The Meaning of Tango*, p. 50.

FOUR: APRIL

1 Louise Bourgeois, *I Have Been to Hell and Back, And Let Me Tell You It was Wonderful*, embroidery on cotton, 1996. *El retorno de lo reprimido (The return of the repressed)*, exhibition, Fundación PROA, La Boca, Buenos Aires, April 2011.

FIVE: MAY

1 L. X. Blonder and J. T. Slevin, 'Emotional dysfunction in Parkinson's disease', *Behavioural Neurology*, 24(3), 2011, pp. 201–17.

2 'Connection between healthy ageing and neurodegenerative disorders', https://cordis.europa.eu/news/rcn/33891/en

3 Simon Armitage, 'Mother, Any Distance', *Book of Matches*, Faber & Faber, London, 1993.

4 Miró J.. 1940. *The Escape Ladder.*; *Joan Miró: The Ladder of Escape* (2011) [Exhibition] Tate Modern, London.

SIX: JUNE

1 C. G. Canning, L. Ada, E. Woodhouse, 'Multiple-task walking training in people with mild to moderate Parkinson's disease: a pilot study', *Clinical Rehabilitation* 22(3), March 2008, pp. 226–33.

2 M. E. Hackney, G. M. Earhart, 'Effects of dance on movement control in Parkinson's disease: a comparison of Argentine tango and American ballroom', *Journal of Rehabilitation Medicine*, 41 (6), May 2009, pp. 475–81.

3 J. R. Hughes, S. G. Bowes, A. L. Leeman et al., 'Parkinsonian abnormality of foot strike: a phenomenon of ageing and/or one responsive to levodopa therapy?', *British Journal of Clinical Pharmacology*, 29 (2), February 1990, pp. 179–86.

4 J. J. Jekka, 'Light-touch contact as a balance aid', *Physical Therapy*, 77 (5), May 1997, pp. 476–87.

5 M. E. Hackney, G. M. Earhart, 'Recommendations for implementing tango classes for persons with Parkinson disease', *American Journal of Dance Therapy*, 32(1), June 2010, pp. 41–52.

SEVEN: JULY

1 Oliver Sacks, 'Kinetic Melody: Parkinson's Disease and Music Therapy', *Musicophilia: Tales of Music and the Brain,* Picador, London, 2007, pp. 248–58.

2 Sophia de Lautour, (2015), 'The Dark History of Canaro's "Poema"', www.so-tango.com/blog/Tango-History-and-Music/thedarkhistoryofcanarospoema (accessed 2 June 2019).

3 Christine Denniston, *The Meaning of Tango: The Story of the Argentinian Dance*, Portico, London, 2007, p. 198.

EIGHT: AUGUST

1 Lloyd Jones, *Here at the End of the World We Learn to Dance,* John Murray, London, 2008.

2 Kristina Olsen, 'My Father's Piano', Take a Break Publishing Company, Venice CA, 1993.

3 Edmund de Waal, *The Hare With Amber Eyes: A Hidden Inheritance*, Chatto & Windus, London, 2010, pp. 250–51.

4 Michael J. Fox, *Lucky Man*, p. 20.

NINE: SEPTEMBER

1 Oliver Sacks, 'Kinetic Melody: Parkinson's Disease and Music Therapy', *Musicophilia: Tales of Music and the Brain,* Picador, London, 2007, p. 258.

2 Kapka Kassabova, *Twelve Minutes of Love: A Tango Story*, Portobello Books, London, 2011

3 Virginia Woolf, *A Room of One's Own*, Hogarth Press, London, 1928.

TEN: OCTOBER

1 William Shakespeare, *King Lear,* Act II, Scene iv.

2 S. Bognar, A. M. DeFaria, C. O'Dwyer et al., 'More than just dancing:

experiences of people with Parkinson's disease in a therapeutic dance program', *Disability and Rehabilitation*, 39 (11), June 2017, pp. 1073–8.

3 Helaine Treitman, *The Embrace of Aging* now available as part of the series, *The Embrace Of*, Visionalist Entertainment Productions, Michigan, 2017 https://theembraceofseries.vhx.tv/

4 Laura Cumming. (2011) 'Joan Miró: The Ladder of Escape – review' *The Observer*, 17 April. Available at https://www.theguardian.com/artanddesign/2011/apr/17/miro-ladder-escape-tate-modern-review (Accessed: 31 May 2019).

ELEVEN: NOVEMBER

1 Joanne Duff et al., 'Making it Happen', *Animated*, Autumn 2011; also see the Dance for PD website, www.danceforparkinsons.org

2 William Shakespeare, Portia, *The Merchant of Venice*, Act IV, Scene i.

3 William Shakespeare, Hotspur, *Henry IV, Part One*, Act III, Scene i.

TWELVE: DECEMBER

1 B. G. DeSylva and Lew Brown (lyrics), Ray Henderson (music), 'Button Up Your Overcoat', performed by Helen Kane, Victor Talking Machine Company, 1929.

2 Johanna Shapiro, 'Illness Narratives: reliability, authenticity and the empathic witness', *Medical Humanities,* 37, July 2011, pp. 68-72.

3 Ibid.

4 John Burnside, 'Pieter Brueghel: Winter Landscape with Skaters and Bird Trap, 1565', *Black Cat Bone,* Jonathan Cape, London, 2011

5 T. S. Eliot, 'The Waste Land', *Selected Poems*, Faber & Faber, London, 1964.

6 T. S. Eliot, 'The Love Song of J. Alfred Prufrock', *Selected Poems*, Faber & Faber, London, 1964.

7 Stevie Smith, 'Not Waving But Drowning' (recording) available at www.poetryarchive.org/search/site/stevie%20smith

8 Julian Barnes, *The Sense of an Ending*, Jonathan Cape, London, 2011, p. 130.

EPILOGUE

1 Information about the English National Ballet Dance for Parkinson's programme is available at www.ballet.org.uk/project/dance-for-parkinsons. My own introduction was via the BBC News item at www.bbc.co.uk/news/uk-england-london-16573752

2 Arthur Miller, *A View from the Bridge, All My Sons*, Penguin, London, 1961.

3 David Leventhal speaking in David Iverson, *Capturing Grace*, Kikim Media, 2014.

4 David Iverson, *Capturing Grace*, Kikim Media, 2014.

APPENDIX: TOUCH: A SHORT STORY

1 www.etymonline.com/word/tango. There is a more detailed discussion in Simon Collier, Artemis Cooper, Maria Susan Azzi et al., *Tango! The Dance, the Song, the Story*, Thames & Hudson, London, 1995, p. 41.

Acknowledgements

My thanks to my first reader, David Connatty, who provided the epigraph; also to readers Emily Bernhard Jackson, Georgia Volioti, Ruth Scurr, Apricot Hulse, Fran Kime and Nicky Beecham; to members of Angles Writing Group in Cambridge for their thoughtful comments and suggestions, and to Marie Vejvodova for her creativity and dedication in making the film *Dancing with Parkinson's*. Thanks also for the music to Michael Lavocah, Michelle McRuiz and James Atkinson, to Colette Paul and Laura Dietz of Anglia Ruskin University, writer Jonathan Taylor, Scilla Dyke of the Royal Academy of Dance, members of English National Ballet's Dance for Parkinson's programme, and Sara Houston of Roehampton University for their interest and encouragement; also to Francis Bertram, Liliana Tolomei, Santiago León and Francesca Halfacree, and to my first tango family, in Cumbria. Thank you, too, to Abby Hoffmann, Nicky Clayton, Robert Shields, Juana Hammond, Peter Sewell, Christine Feig, Jay Weatherly, Aysel Deniz, Ange Vete, Derek Smith, Mel Driver, Jan Hurst and Jan Green, and to Roger Barker and the team at the

Cambridge Centre for Brain Repair, in particular Romina Vuono. Thanks also to Ray Harper, Adam Carpenter, Felicity Devonshire, Fay Roberts, Rowena Whitehead, Tom Ling and John Betmead, Belona Greenwood, Nicolo Chiodarelli, Katy Bailey and Lewis Jones. A massive thank you to the hundreds who gave their support during the crowdfunding process, with a special mention for Clare Crossman and for Louise Ells and her Aunt Em. Finally, thanks to friends, family and all at Cambridge Tango, and to my two long-suffering co-conspirators, John and Ellie, without whom there would be no story to tell.

A Note on the Author

After thirty years as an English teacher in London, the north of England and Mexico City, Kate Swindlehurst moved to Cambridge, where she gained a distinction in the MA in creative writing at Anglia Ruskin University and won an Arts Council Escalator Award to work on a novel about Argentina's disappeared. As writer in residence at Cambridge University Botanic Garden, she produced a short-story collection, *Writing the Garden*. Her novel *The Station Master*, based on our responses to the refugee crisis, won the 2017 Adventures in Fiction Spotlight competition for debut novelists and was shortlisted for the Caledonia Novel Award in 2019.

kateswindlehurst.com

Unbound is the world's first crowdfunding publisher, established in 2011.

We believe that wonderful things can happen when you clear a path for people who share a passion. That's why we've built a platform that brings together readers and authors to crowdfund books they believe in – and give fresh ideas that don't fit the traditional mould the chance they deserve.

This book is in your hands because readers made it possible. Everyone who pledged their support is listed below. Join them by visiting unbound.com and supporting a book today.

Ruth Ainley
Martin Anderssohn
Rebecca Armour
Deborah Arnander
Andrew Aston
Karen Attwood
Sharon Baird
Louise Baker
Sally Beckwith
Nicky Beecham
Ninah Beliavsky

Kaddy Benyon
The Big Weekend Coffee
 Crowd
Elaine Bishop
Stefan Blaser
Anna Blume
Maxine Bodell
Sandra Borszcz
Izzy Bowles
Danny Brunton
Norma Caira

Cat Campbell
Karen Cannon
Adam Carpenter
Jan Casey
Leigh Chambers
Alix Chancellor
Nancy Chinnery
Norma Clarke
Di Clay
Nick Clay
Nicky Clayton
Andy Clements
Susannah Clements
Nick Clifton-Welker
Judith Clute
Clara Collart
John Connatty
Irene Costa
Sally Cowens
Cresset BioMolecular
   Discovery Limited
Clare Crossman
Jocelyn Curtis
Anna D'Andrea
Mona Melicia De Silva
Joy Dee
Stephen Delaney
Richard Devonshire
Laura Dietz
Nicola Dodd

Dodie
Lisa Donald
Dot & Wimp
Michael Doyle
Alex Elbro
Carole Ellison
M.J. Fahy
Peter Faulkner
Theresa Feetenby
Christine Feig
Stef Ferrucci
David Foley
Luigi Formisano
Rose Foster
Louise Foxcroft
Melissa Fu
John Gale
Guinevere Glasfurd
Miranda Gold
Miranda Gomperts
Jan Green
Susan Griffith
Eryl Griffiths
Katy Guest
Francesca Halfacree
Jilly Hall
Lynne Hall
Lucy Hamilton
Di Hampton
Penny Hancock

Catherine Harlow

Ray Harper

Kate Hauxwell

Milo Hawker

Gloria Heilbronn

Britta Heinemeyer

Angèle Hélène

Penny Hemingway

Penny Henderson

Martin & June Henry

Ceri Higgins

Sue Hill

Robin Hinson

Penny Hodgkinson

Tim Holt-Wilson

Raymond Honeyman

Antonia Honeywell

Ana Höpping

Philip Hoser

Sara Houston

Mandy Howarth

Carrie Jo Howe

Paul Hughes

Catherine Hunt

Megan Hunter

Jan Hurst

Oliver Jackson

Jenny Jarvis

Brenna John

Martin Johnson

Christine Jones

Matthew Jones

Helle Jørgensen

Lizz Kendon

Ann Kennedy Smith

Dan Kieran

Fran Kime

Carole Kirby

David & Michele Lambert

Christy Lane

Paul Lausell

Madeline Lees

Lenabellina

Laura Lou Levy

Sari Lievonen

Chris Limb

Joanne Limburg

Christine Lloyd

Nat Lund

Dr Amy Mallett

Lara Martyn

Louis Martyn

Robert Mason

Elizabeth McCaig

Sabrina McCready

Di McEvoy-Robinson

Marie McGinley

Iain Mcphee

Rosie Meikle

Kaarina Meyer

Godfrey & Honor Meynell

The Michael J Foxtrotters

John Mitchinson

Azadeh Moaveni

Renée Molho

Jane Monson

Cathy Moore

Anthony Morgan

Nicola M Morgan

Bob Murray

Alexandra Murrell

Carlo Navato

Lasse Nielsen

Eileen Norman

Kerry O'Connell

Cathal O'Luanaigh

Kristina Olsen

Yoko Oshima

David Palfreyman

Sue Palfreyman

Libby Parker

Melanie Parker

Geoff Patterson

Colette Paul

Miranda Perdja

Hugo Perks

Margaret Phillips

Justin Pollard

Hugh Pollock

Jennifer Pollock

Vanessa Price

Nancy Priest

Jude Pullman

Niall Quinn

Adam Quinney

Linda Quinney

Susana Quintanilha

In memory of my Aunt,
   Emily Rawlence Bilmes

Jean Rees

Katie Reynolds

Alyson Rheinbach

Cora Roberts

Richard Robinson

Helen Rose

Jamie Rose

Alex Ruczaj

Gary Ruggera

Ellie Rush

Bridget Salmon

Jane Sanders

Wendy Saville

Katriona Scoffin

James Scott

Hilary Seaward

Patricia Seguin

Peter Sewell

Laurence Shapiro

Philip Shaw

Lucy Sheerman

Robert Shields

Rifat Siddiqui

Debbie Simpson

Fiona Simpson

Jude Simpson

Mary Skelley

Cecille Slish

Robert Small

Derek Smith

Geoff Smith

Professor David Spendlove

Ralph Sperring

Valerie Spotswood

Michelle Spring

Brigitte Squire

Leo Stickley

Sarah Story

Susan Stuart

Bridget Sumsion

Zoe Swenson-Wright

Jack Swindlehurst

Jonathan & Maria Taylor

Matthew Taylor

Adam & Lorna Tinworth

Heather Tipler

John Tomlinson

Maggi Toner-Edgar

Lynn Travis

Norma Turvill

Stephen Twist

Jernej Ule

Tony Vanderheyden

Marie Vejvodová

Georgia Volioti

Ruth Wade

Jo Walker

Linda Warnes

Maurice Watts

Jay Weatherly

Ann Williamson

Catherine Williamson

Marlene Williamson

Max Wind-Cowie

Kurt Wintersteiner

Julie Winyard

John Wood

Tim Wood

Peter Woolnough

Colin and Rachel Wright

Ben Wylie

Barbara Young